SCISSORS AND COMB
HAIRCUTTING

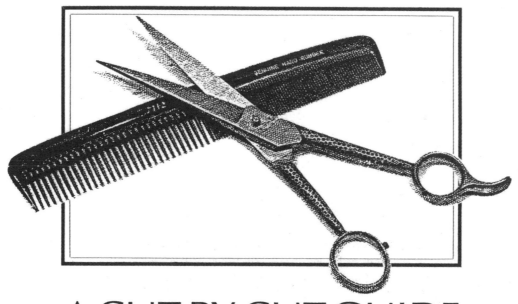

A CUT-BY-CUT GUIDE

WRITTEN AND ILLUSTRATED BY
BOB OHNSTAD

1

copyright © 2012 by Robert E. Ohnstad

24 22 20 18 16 14   10 9 8 7 6 5 4 3 2 1

Printed in the United States of America

Library of Congress Cataloging in Publication Data

Ohnstad, Bob, 1941 -

   Scissors and comb haircutting

   Includes index.
   1.Haircutting. I. Title.
TT970.037   1985   646.7'242   84-90072
ISBN 0-916819-01-9 (soft)

Published by
You Can Publishing
P.O. Box 11400
Minneapolis, Minnesota 55411

Visit our website: www.howtocuthair.com

SCISSOR AND COMB HAIRCUTTING
a cut-by-cut guide

CONTENTS

INTRODUCTION

HISTORY. This second edition is the eighth printing and first revision of "Scissors and Comb Haircutting." I first got the idea to write this book after teaching some friends how to give haircuts they could feel good about. Then in the late 1970s I was hospitalized with pneumonia. As I waited to learn what was wrong with me, the idea of writing a book came to me again. Three things contributed to my book writing decision: I had acquired a variety of skills from twenty (now fifty) years of haircutting with many different barbers; a four-year teaching degree gave me another set of skills; and finally those friends who became haircutters with my help. Another factor was the belief I could write my book in a few months. Five years later the first printing was in my hands. I needed much help to get this book done--editing, cover design, more editing, typesetting, still more editing, support from my wife and family, friends, customers, parents and more. This book would still be a dream without them.

MY APPROACH. There are many ways to cut and care for hair. My approach is a simple one: I give my customers a precision haircut every month or two that makes their hair look good all the time with just shampoo and towel-dry haircare. These are basic haircuts that have been popular for many decades--people like them year after year because they're so easy to maintain. To top it off, reasonable prices keeps more money in my customer's pocket. If I needed a haircut, I would look for the kind of shop my daughter and I operate.

HOW TO USE THE BOOK. Professionals and students can read any part of the book and gain worthwhile how-to. Those new to haircutting should read the book cover to cover. One reading builds confidence and destroys the myth that only a few creative types can cut hair. Beginners should give it another reading or two, and then use the book as a cut-by-cut guide when they begin haircutting.

Thanks for letting me share my passion for haircutting with you. Expect to have fun.

WELCOME TO PEOPLE-PLEASING PRECISION HAIRCUTTING!

***

The best effect of any book is that it excites the reader to self activity.   Thomas Carlyle
A good teacher is one who makes himself progressively unnecessary.   Anonymous

CHAPTER 1 ABOUT HAIR

1.1 CLOSE-UP OF A HAIR

One of the more amazing things in our world is the snowflake. Each of those little frozen crystals are a one-of-a-kind creation. Despite the uniqueness, similarities are seen from one flake to the next. So it is with heads of hair--no two are exactly alike, but similarities exist from one to the next.

This first section's examination of hair is concerned with things common to all hair; later sections describe different qualities that make every head of hair unique. To begin, these four terms are used to describe a hair from one end to the other.

A. Four Parts of a Hair

1. End: The oldest part of the hair is also called the tip.
2. Hair shaft: The visible part of a hair.
3. Root: The part of the hair that exists below the skin.
4. Bulb: The little bump found at the bottom of a growing hair. This newest part of the hair is hard to see, but your finger tips can feel it when a hair falls out or is pulled out.

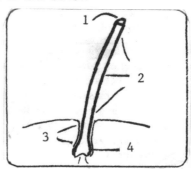

The root and bulb are parts of a hair not seen while hair is growing; they are surrounded by the complex growth "factory" we examine next.

B. The Follicle

My dictionary defines a hair follicle as the sheath that surrounds the lower, subcutaneous part of the hair. That doesn't say much about the busy nature of a follicle.)

My description is more detailed: A follicle is that part of the skin surrounding the hair root and bulb, and it produces the different cells that make up a growing hair. The follicle is about 1/4 inch deep and. includes these parts:

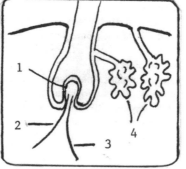

1. Papilla: The site of hair cell production.
2. Blood vessel: Brings nourishment to papilla.
3. Nerve supply: The growth cycle regulator.
4. Sebaceous glands: Produces natural oil.

The small cone-shaped elevation at the bottom of the hair follicle is the papilla. With its blood and nerve supply, the papilla is the source of pain you feel when a hair is pulled out prematurely--the bulb grows around the papilla and tugs at it when a hair receives pullout pressure. The nerve supply sends the papilla's pain message to the brain, but more important, it acts as an on-and-off switch to control the different stages of hair growth (described later in this chapter). The blood vessel brings the nutrients needed to keep the papilla humming along with its cell-production activities. The sebaceous glands produce a natural oil called sebum. This oil travels from the gland, through a duct to the hair root or up to the scalp; eventually the oil coats all the hair as it journeys up the hair shaft to the tip of the hair. Sebaceous glands don't produce much until puberty, and their production usually slows after age 45 to 50.

C. The Different Layers of a Hair

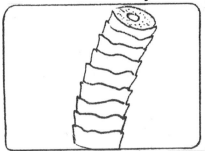 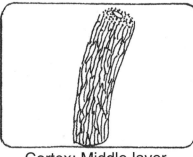 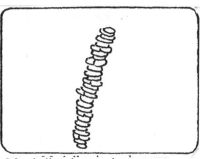

Cuticle: Outside layer   Cortex: Middle layer   Medulla: Inner layer

A hair has two or three layers depending on how thick it is. Each hair has a **cuticle layer** composed of hard, round, tubular cells. These outside armor cells protect the softer, inner layers. If the hair is in a healthy condition the cuticle cells lie flat and overlap each other. In this state, the outside layer can perform its primary function of protection. An added bonus is a healthy-looking sheen.

If the cuticle layer becomes damaged the overlapping part of the cell will curl up. This condition diffuses light, making the hair appear dull. When the cuticle gets to this state, the soft cortex layer is exposed and damage such as split ends and hair breakage is likely.

The **cortex layer** consists of long, spindle-shaped cells that lie parallel to the hair shaft's length. These soft cells contain melanin, the color-giving pigment. Melanin combines with air bubbles in the cortex layer to give hair its many shades of brown, blond, black, and red (melanin is absent in white hair and fairly sparse in grey hair).

The third layer of cells, which may not exist on small diameter hair, is **the medulla.** This innermost layer is composed of soft, coin-shaped cells stacked on top of each other in an irregular manner.

D. Chemical Composition of Hair

Hair is composed of keratin, a protein substance also found in the skin, finger nails, and toe nails. The approximate chemical makeup of hair is: 50% carbon, 20% oxygen, 20% nitrogen, 5% sulfur, and 5% hydrogen. Because of hair's nitrogen content, it is a welcome, but slow-to-decompose addition to the compost pile or garden.

E. Hair's Function

Those hairs on your head are not just an adornment, or a nuisance to be endured. They function as a cushion against blows to that delicate brain, and as an effective temperature insulator. In winter a large part of a person's body heat is lost through the top of the head; a bald head loses body heat much faster than a full head of hair. In the warm months, hair serves to insulate against the sun's heat. Other things being equal, a bald person will suffer a heat stroke much sooner than a person with abundant hair.

1.2 NUMBER OF HAIRS AND RATE OF GROWTH

The numbers of hairs on a head, and the growth rate, are two hair factors that help make every head of hair unique. An average adult head has 120 square inches of hair-growing surface (the scalp) with a little less than 1,000 hairs per square inch. Hair color makes a difference: Blondes average 120,000 hairs on their heads; brown and black-haired people have about 110,000; and redheads usually have 95,000, give or take a few thousand. With many exceptions to these averages, these numbers still hold fairly true.

The number of active hair follicles on our heads slowly decreases throughout one's life span, and males have more of a decrease than females. Whereas deer grow new hair follicles throughout their lives, we have to be satisfied with the follicles we get at birth. How fast the hair grows has a relationship to the hair's diameter and color. Finer, lighter-colored hair usually grows 3/8 inch a month. For the rest of us, those hairs can sprout as much as 3/4 inch, however the average is 1/2 inch per month. Darker hair usually grows faster than lighter, coarser hair faster than finer. Gray hairs seem to flourish a little faster than the colored hair they replace.

The growth rate is the same for each of those 100,000 thread-like objects on the head. While the rate may speed up a little for gray hairs, and it's usually slower for children in their first year or two, the rate otherwise remains constant throughout our life span.

1.3 HAIR TYPES

Hair type is another factor that contributes to the uniqueness of every head of hair. The last chapter describes how this subject can get a little muddled by some hair conditions, but here we examine the four terms used to describe this characteristic of hair.

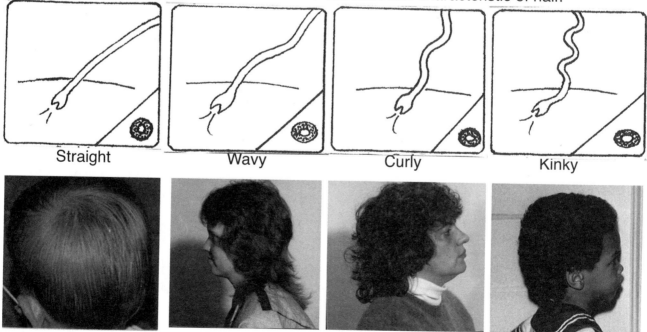

Straight   Wavy   Curly   Kinky

These drawings and photographs illustrate the differences between the various types of hair. The cross sections of hair (in the lower right corners of the drawings) show straight hair is the roundest, and kinky hair is the flattest. Note that the curlier hair is, the more it grows up and out from the scalp, whereas straighter hair grows out at less of an angle and lies closer to the head. The angle of growth from the scalp leads to the next subject.

1.4 HAIR GRAIN

From experience I've found that only a minority of barbers or hairstylists, and virtually no customers know that every head of hair has a unique hair grain. You need a thorough understanding of hair grain because this factor determines the lying direction of straighter types of hair. As a result, hair grain makes a major contribution to the final appearance of your haircuts. Also, the hair grain has a big impact on the way you use the tools during the haircutting process.

This hair phenomena, sometimes called the hair-growth pattern, has to do with the direction the hair grows from the head, and the fact that an individual hair grows out from the scalp in the same general direction as its neighbors.

Hair doesn't grow out from the head in a willy-nilly manner. 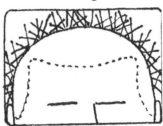 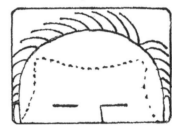 Hair has a fairly uniform way of growing from the head that reflects its hair grain.

A. My Best Hair-grain Explanation

When I explain hair grain to my customers, I use the example of a dog with short straight hair. Run your hand through the hair on its back, from tail to head: The hair stands on end for a moment, then lies down again, returning to its natural lying position toward the tail. The hair lies in this particular way because a dog's coat has a definite hair-grain pattern--the angle the hairs grow out from the skin is quite uniform from one hair to the next.

We share this characteristic with our canine friends. Whether it's the tresses on our head, beard hair, or other body hair, our hair grows out from the skin in a **definite pattern.** While there are gradual changes in the hair's lying direction (and sometimes abrupt changes), for the most part individual hairs grow out from the skin in the same direction as their neighbors.

If hair grew straight up, the concept of hair grain would not exist. 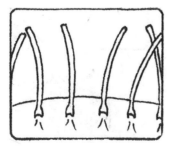 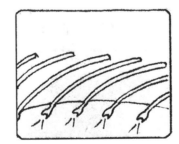 Hair emerges at an angle, with its neighbors having the same angle. Hence the **pattern** is created.

***

Don't talk unless you can improve the silence. Vermont proverb

He labors vainly who endeavors to please everyone. Latin proverb

B. Two Basic Types of Hair grain

Every head of hair has its own unique grain, its way of growing out of the scalp. Despite this uniqueness, you'll find two basic hair grain patterns describe nearly all heads of hair. These two types mainly focus on how the hair grows on the sides.

• **Type 1 hair grain**: The side hair grows downward, toward the ears.

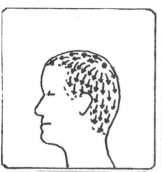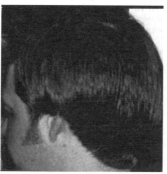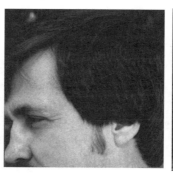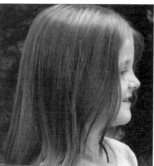

About 40 percent of people have this pattern. Normally this hair grain is found on straight-haired people.

• **Type 2 hair grain**: The side hair grows toward the back of the head.

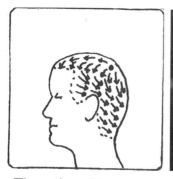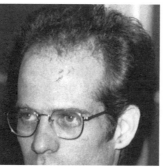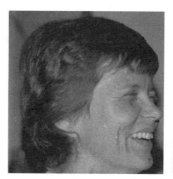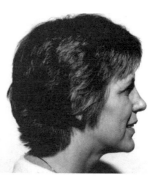

The other 60 percent of the world's population has this pattern. Type 2 hair grain is usually associated with wavier, curly, and kinky hair.

A common feature of the Type 2 hair grain is the ducktail neckline. With a Type 1 grain, the hair at the neck normally grows straight down, while a Type 2 usually grows in a pattern of curves and whorls at the nape of the neck, just like a duck's tail.

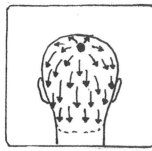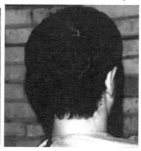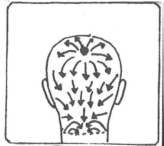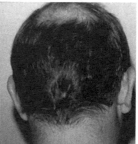

Type 1.   Type 2 and the ducktail neck grain.

Chapter 6 has more examples of this common neck grain pattern.

C. The Cowlick

Now we go to the heart of the matter, the cowlick. Despite popular opinion, the cowlick is much more than an ornery tuft of hair that annoys some people. To begin unraveling this subject, you should know that every person's crown region (the upper back part of the head) has one cowlick, and on a small percentage of heads, you'll find two back there, and maybe even discover an extra cowlick on the front top hairline. This hair phenomena is the starting point that establishes the pattern of the hair grain. Put another way, the cowlick is the center of the hair grain.

I like to describe the cowlick as if it were the axle of a bicycle wheel. The hair in the immediate vicinity of the cowlick is like the spokes of the wheel--just as the spokes go out and away from the axle, the hair also goes out and away from the cowlick.

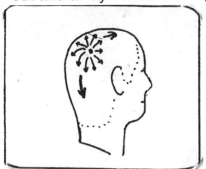 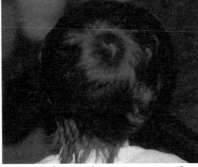 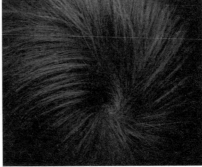

The hair grows away from the center point, the cowlick

Wherever you find the cowlick in the crown region (in the center area or off-center, toward the front or in a lower position), the hair grows out and away from it--down toward the bottom of the neck, and forward toward the front of the top of the head. It always happens that the hair grain is directed toward the front on top, however slightly different growth patterns depend on where the cowlick is positioned. If the cowlick is on the left, you usually find this hair-grain pattern

Left-side cowlick and its normal hair grain.

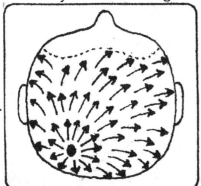 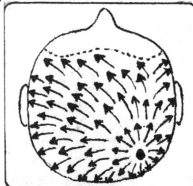

A right-side cowlick usually has this hair grain pattern.

You will find this unusual reversal of the pattern on about 5% of heads.

Left-side cowlick with a reversed hair grain.

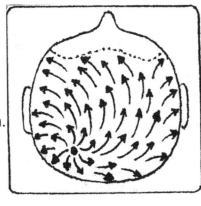 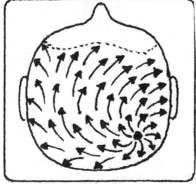

Right-side cowlick with this unusual hair-grain.

When the cowlick is located in the center of the crown region, three different hair grain patterns are possible:

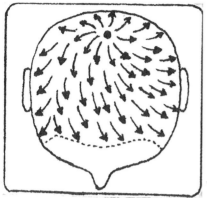 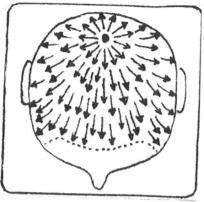 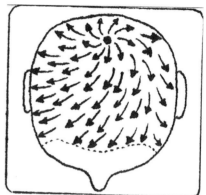

The cowlick's position and the resulting hair-grain pattern, contributes to the uniqueness of every head of hair

D. Cowlick Confusion

How can every head of hair have at least one cowlick, yet so few people know this basic hair fact? The reason behind this befuddlement has to do with how longer and curlier hair is able to hide that little cowlick.

Long hair. Although straight hair is the hair type most affected by the hair-grain and cowlick, longer straight hair gets heavy and bends downward because of its weight and the force of gravity. Because this bending happens near the roots, it's common for the cowlick region to be covered over by long, bent hairs. When this hair is cut on the short side, the surplus weight is gone and the bending no longer occurs. The hair lies the way it wants (in all directions away from the cowlick) and that cowlick is easily seen.

Curly and kinky hair. This kind of hair hides the cowlick because it grows out from the scalp like coiled springs:

Curly and kinky hair coils out and away from the head. 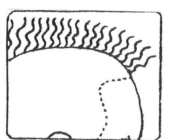 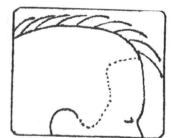 In contrast, straighter hair lies close to the head.

Straight hair lies down, and that shows more of the hair shaft making it easy to see the hair's grain and cowlick. Curlier hair results in a head of hair where all you see is the ends--the hair-grain and cowlick are well camouflaged. If this hair is cut quite short (less than an inch) the hair-grain and cowlick can be seen.

When curly and kinky hair is cut short enough so that the first upward bend is cut off, the hair-grain and cowlick shows itself. Once the hair has grown another 1/2 inch or so, it bends upward again and "springs" out from the scalp, and the cowlick is back in a state of hiding. With that extra half inch of length, this kind of hair can be combed or brushed in any direction.

You will learn in Chapter 6 that wavy, curly, and kinky hair types can be cut to just about any length. Straighter kinds of hair tend to have one best length.

E. The Standup-Cowlick Problem

Sometimes the hair grain and cowlick hide. Occasionally the hair grain's center point makes itself most visible. I'm talking about that stubborn tuft of hair that stands out from the rest of the hair in the crown region. This wild hair problem only happens with straight or wavy hair. The curlier types of hair grow out from the scalp all over the head, so all the hair ends blend--they all stand up, so no crown region hairs stand out from the rest. There are four possible causes for cowlick hairs standing on end, but two or more of these causes may combine to make a little tuft into a major eruption. We begin with the most common source of the problem.

Wrong combing direction. Whenever hair that wants to lie away from the cowlick is combed or brushed in a direction against the hair's natural lying inclination, you'll have standup problems. Most commonly, this occurs with the hair that grows from the crown-area cowlick toward the top front hairline: When the hair lies the way it wants, there's no standup problem.

Hair is combed with the grain, toward the front.

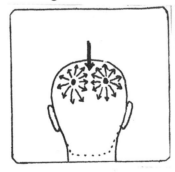
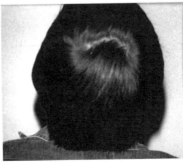

Hair is combed toward the back, which is against the grain.

Fight the hair's natural way of lying and you'll have standup problems

Twin cowlicks. About 10 percent of people exhibit the hair-grain phenomena known as twin or double cowlicks. Two center points in the crown region doesn't always make the hair stick out back there, but on about a third of these people the hair between the cowlicks wants to stand on end, particularly if it is cut too short. The rule is: The less space between twin cowlicks (1 1/2 inches or less), the more the hair growing between the cowlicks wants to stand on end. The consequence of this rule is that you have to leave the hair longer so it will bend and lie down with the other hair around it.

The hair wants to stand out at the clash-point between the cowlicks.

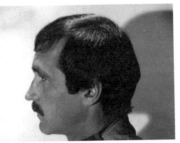

The line you see between the two cowlicks is a natural parting of the hair created by separation of the hairs that lie toward the front of the head, and those lying toward the neck.

• **Low cowlick**. About 10 percent of cowlicks are found in a lower-than-normal position.

***

If fifty million people say a foolish thing, it is still a foolish thing.   Anatole France

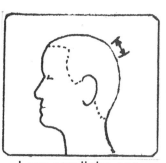
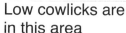

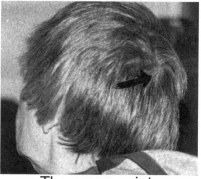

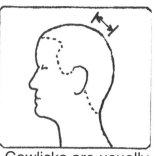

Low cowlicks are
in this area

The arrow points
at the cowlick

Cowlicks are usually
in this area

The low cowlick produces a standout problem because the hair that wants to lie toward the top front of the head has an uphill battle against the forces of gravity.

The arrows point to the uphill area where the hair wants to lie toward the front of the head.

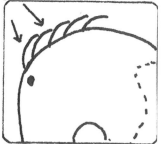

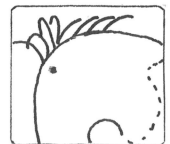

But gravity pulls that hair down toward the back of the head. When hair doesn't lie the way it wants, standout hair is the rule. The chapter on determining the right length describes an easy remedy.

•**Cut too short**. Fewer than 5 percent of people have a single cowlick in the crown region that has to be left on the longer side. With these people you find that your best estimate for hair length on top of the head was right on the mark, but you end up with a few hairs standing on end in the cowlick area. This fairly rare problem proves cutting hair is not 100 percent predictable; you may be a bit off on your length calculations when you come across a stubborn cowlick like this: Just leave it a little longer the next time you cut it. Standout hair in the cowlick or anywhere is not a problem with people who wear stand-up (spiked) styles that have become more common, but,costly products are required to get the hair standing on end.

F. The Exceptional Hair grain

Nine times out of ten, the hair grain on one side of the head is a mirror image of the hair grain on the other side. Occasionally it's slightly different; however, one head in a hundred will differ a lot: You may find one side growing straight down, while the other side grows toward the back of the head.

The center of the hair grain (the cowlick) is a fairly routine matter, but recently I came across a first: I was giving a haircut to a man who surprised me with his two extra cowlicks. Each was an inch up from the neck's bottom hairline, about two inches apart, and the "knowledge bump" (located where the spine meets the skull), was directly between the two cowlicks. I've seen people with an extra cowlick at the bottom edge of the neck hair, but never a cowlick so high up into the back hair--and then to see a pair of them! What next? The "snowflake" nature of hair keeps this an always-interesting, sometimes-surprising craft. Just when you think you've seen it all, you meet a head of hair that proves you wrong.

G. Checking the Hair grain

To determine if you are dealing with a Type 1 or Type 2 hair grain, comb through the hair and look closely at the direction of the hair coming out of the scalp.

Comb through the hair in an upward direction on the sides, and look closely at the base of the hairs that fall from the comb as it moves up through the hair.

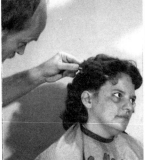 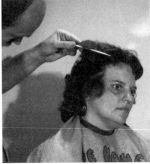 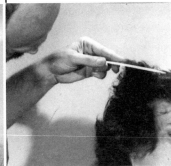

Note the direction of the first 1/2 inch of hair coming out of the follicles: This is the part of the hair most influenced by the hair grain. Longer hair bends downward because of weight and gravity--if you look at the hair beyond the 1/2 inch point, you are likely to see bent hair that gives a false reading.

Use this upward combing and close inspection to check the back hair for a ducktail neckline. On the top, comb in a front-to-back direction to check for cowlick(s) and for the direction (to the left or right) that the top wants to lie.

Straighter hair shows its hair grain farther from the follicle than do curlier varieties. This means you need to look extra close at the newest part of the hair shafts on wavier and curlier hair.

H. Hair grain and Genetics

In my first years of barbering, my services were limited to men and boys. Since I started giving haircuts to all the members of the family, I have a better picture of the influence genetics has on a person's hair. Now I feel safe in saying the hair grain (as well as the other major hair characteristics) is determined by genes. The genetic influence is quite noticeable in any family, but it was especially obvious on my identical twin customers. The genetic influence on hair usually comes from Mom or Dad, but sometimes you have to look to grandparents or great grandparents.

I. Beard grain

Whiskers lay in these three general patterns:

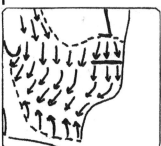 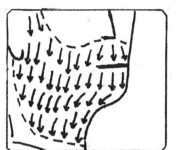 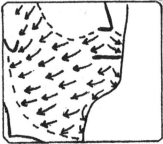

Typical.   Two common exceptions.

The rule is: Whiskers generally grow downward except on the lower half or two-thirds of the neck where the hairs grow upward, and then off to the sides of the neck. There are two common exceptions: (1) The neck hair grows down with no upward or reverse grain. (2) The hair grows somewhat downward, but mainly toward the sides of the neck. You can easily check out the grain on a freshly shaved face: Run your fingers over the shaved area--if it feels smooth you're going with the grain, if it feels like sandpaper, you're going against it.

Men who shave with a safety razor or the old-time straightedge razor, usually have some notion of the beard's grain. If their shaving blade is directed against the beard's grain, they will get an extra close--sometimes too close--shave that can leave the skin irritated, and even cause ingrown hairs, infections, and rashes. If the blade travels with the direction of the grain, the result is a less close, but more comfortable shave.

J. Hair Grain High Points

This section on hair grain contains a lot of information. It's important stuff because hair grain has a big impact on the hair's appearance and, as shown in later chapters, on how you handle tools. To recap, these are the major points:

• **Unique, yet similar.** While the hair grain contributes to a head of hair's uniqueness, nearly everyone's hair can be classified as having a Type 1 or Type 2 hair grain.

• **Permanent.** The grain of the hair is something a person is born with, and it's as unchangeable as fingerprints.

•**The hair grain is boss.** The grain of the hair determines the lying direction of straight or wavy hair. This natural force on the hair diminishes when the hair is longer than 2 to 3 inches. Then the hair can bend, and its weight, plus gravity, has an impact on its lying direction.

• **Curly-hair characteristics.** It is difficult to see the hair grain on wavier and curlier hair because they grow out from the scalp. This hair is less affected by the hair grain because it can usually lie in any direction, if it's cut short enough. As it grows longer, curly hair will return to its stand-out-from-the-head nature.

• **The hair grain's center point.** Everyone has one cowlick in the crown region of their head; some have two. When a cowlick stands on end its usually because the hair in that area isn't lying the way the hair grain wants it to lay.

1.5 TEXTURE OF HAIR

The texture of the hair refers to the thickness or thinness of individual hairs. The diameter of the hairs on the head can be as large as 1/100 inch or as small as 1/500 inch. For purposes of classification, the terms fine, medium, and coarse are used. Fine hair tends to be lighter and coarse hair usually has a darker color. Medium-textured hair can be any color.

Assume that each of these hairs is two inches long.

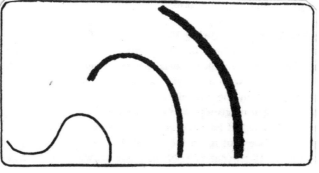

Fine   Medium   Coarse

As this drawing indicates, fine hair is the softest, most bendable of the three.

As chapter 6 points out, texture is the major factor in deciding what is the best length for straighter types of hair.

Age has an impact on the hair's diameter. At birth we have the finest-textured hair; by the time we are in puberty, our hair has expanded to its maximum diameter; and when hair turns gray or white, it's common to have a coarser texture that may not lay as well as the colored hair it has replaced.

The whole head of hair can be referred to as thick or thin. When hair is described this way, it's not about the hair's texture, it's a matter of the number of hairs per square inch.

1.6 THE HAIR GROWTH CYCLE

A. The Three-Stage Cycle

Most people are not aware that their hair maintains a steady process of growth, resting, and shedding, and then the follicle starts a new growth cycle. Many believe when a hair falls out it's gone forever, making them one step closer to baldness. This notion is way off the mark.

An individual hair's life cycle has three different stages to go through. First is the **anagen** stage or the growth part of the cycle. A hair grows at a continuous rate for as little as two years for some people, to as long as six or more years for others. How long a person's hair remains in its growing stage depends some on age, but a lot on genetics: (1) As a teenager you experience a longer anagen stage than you do in your later years, (2) the genes your parents passed onto you make all the difference between a short growing season and a long one. With the second part of the cycle, the **catagen** stage, the papilla stops its production of hair cells. This shutting-down stage lasts for as long as a month, and results in the follicle shrinking. The next step in the cycle is the **telogen** stage. In this part, the hair growth factory rests. When the follicle has stopped shrinking, the mature hair can hang around for another 2-3 months. During this time, the shrunken follicle holds onto the hair unless it is dislodged by shampooing or brushing. At the end of this stage, the follicle resumes its normal shape and it's time for another anagen stage. The papilla starts production again, and a new hair starts to grow. Now the old hair either falls out or is pulled out, or the newly emerging hair pushes out the old hair. In a couple of weeks, the new hair appears from the follicle, and grows for another 2 to 6 years.

At any time, over 85 percent of your hairs are in the long-lasting anagen stage of the growth cycle, while the remainder of the hairs on your head are in either the catagen or telogen stages. This continuous cycle results in a daily shedding of 50 to 150 hairs. You'll always lose hair. The key to having a healthy growing head of hair is to keep on replacing the "bailed-out" hairs with new ones, and to keep that anagen stage coming back for more.

B. Long Versus Short Growing Heads of Hair

Two different people could let their hair grow for five years without any haircutting; one may end up with waist-length or longer hair, while the other's locks only grow to about 6 inches below the neck. This difference is caused by the rate of hair growth per month, and the length of the anagen or growth part of the cycle.

Eventually a head of hair reaches the point at which it won't get any longer. This does not mean the overall head of hair stops growing (remember, over 85 percent of your hairs are growing all the time). It does mean the oldest, longest hairs on the head have finally reached the catagen stage, soon to be followed by the telogen, the resting-and-fallout stage. These longest hairs that eventually fall out are continuously being replaced by other long hairs that are approaching the end of their growth cycle. The length of the bottom edge remains constant, but the majority of hairs continue growing.

1.7 THE DIFFERENT KINDS OF HAIR LOSS

The three stages of hair growth result in a daily shedding of about 100 hairs. If the daily discard exceeds this amount in a big way, then something out of the ordinary is probably happening. A number of causes create abnormal loss of hair--some are permanent, some are temporary, and some are not what they appear to be.

A. Confusion About Hair loss
Some of the things we do to our hair results in what appears to abnormal hair loss:
• **Hair breakage**. Some people, especially those with fine-textured hair, can suffer hair damage that results in the hair breaking off. There are a number of possible causes, but chemical processing (permanents, hair straighteners) and too much swimming in chlorinated water are the two common ones. You can easily determine breakage by examining hairs that come from shampooing or brushing. If these hairs don't have a "bump" on one end (the bulb), the hair has broken off. If you can feel the bulb, it's not breakage.
Infrequent shampooing. If people shampoo once a week, they will find much more hair in the tub or sink than if they shampooed daily. Shampooing and brushing dislodges hairs that are in the telogen stage. If these hairs are not dislodged, eventually they fall out or are pushed out by new growth. If you shampoo weekly, you will have 168 hours of telogen stage hairs waiting to be dislodged, while daily shampooing produces only 24 hours of this natural shedding. Infrequent shampooing makes it appear as if you are losing a lot of hair, but really you're not (unless that scalp gets to the "crusty" stage described in section C-2 on the next page).

B. Temporary Hair loss: Six Possibilities
Anyone can experience extraordinary hair loss in a fairly short period of time. Dealing with any of the possible causes always takes time (and patience) before the normal growth cycle resumes and those lost hairs are replaced. The different causes are:
1. Physical stress. Severe fever, major surgery, shock, etc.
2. Emotional stress. Any extra stressful environment or way of living can do it.
3. Blessed event. Because of the hormonal changes that happen at childbirth, significant hair loss can be expected.
4. Drugs. Using cortisones and amphetamines will do it. Many lose hair after stopping the use of birth control pills.
5. Hormonal disorders. Particularly those associated with the thyroid or sex glands.
6. Diet deficiencies. Without protein, the follicles go on vacation. Even vitamin or mineral deficiencies can cause it.

C. Permanent Hair loss: The Causes

When an individual hair follicle permanently stops production, the shutdown is usually a result of inherited tendencies, or it is caused by something you do or don't do.

1.**Genetic heritage**. Your genetic heritage is, by far, the most important factor in going bald. When it is genetically the right time for that growth factory to shut down, that's exactly what happens despite your best efforts to the contrary--it's all beyond your control. Permanent hair loss (alopecia) is a part of aging: Taken as a group, about thirty percent of thirty-year-olds will experience significant hair loss. For every one year increase in age we see a 1percent increase in the number of bald men, i.e., 40 percent of forty-year-olds and 60 percent of sixty-year-olds will have lost a significant amount of their top hair.

This shutting down of hair follicles is tied to your hormonal system. At a genetically determined moment the male hormone, testosterone, accumulates in the blood vessel going to the papilla, shutting it down permanently. The only things that stop this process for men (it's called male-pattern baldness) are castration or taking large doses of the female hormone, estrogen. Ignoring the first possibility, the second option works but it has the side effects of breast and hip growth, and facial hair loss.

Permanent hair loss in women is also associated with the male hormone; however, it is thought that because a woman's hormonal system produces only 25 percent of the testosterone that a man's system does, she loses much less hair than he. In both cases, the testosterone is to blame. For women, hair loss of this type usually occurs during menopause. Then the estrogen production is slowing, but testosterone levels remain constant, producing a limited hair loss. Estrogen hormone therapy may be considered a solution, but risks include the possibility of blood clotting, strokes, and cancer.

2. **Abuse**. People permanently lose their hair when their genetics say it time to go. However, abuse has to do with what we do (or not do) that can speed up the process. Unlike genetics, we have some control over what happens to our hair, so it's covered in the next chapter on healthy haircare.

***

The real purpose of books is to trap the mind into doing its own thinking.

Christopher Morley

No one is useless in this world who lightens the burdens of another.   Charles Dickens

There is no higher religion than human service. To work for the common good is the greatest creed.

Albert Schweitzer

It's what we value-not what we have-that makes us rich.   Dr. J. Harold Smith

Those who need help are not near as needy as those who refuse to give it.   Anonymous

Selfishness is at the root of virtually every hurtful, evil-minded act ever committed.

Unknown

Repay evil with good and you deprive the evildoer of all the pleasures of his wickedness.

Leo Tolstoy

Honesty and transparency make you vulnerable. Be honest and transparent anyway.

Mother Teresa

CHAPTER 2 HEALTHY HAIRCARE

You can give people outstanding haircuts, but if your customer doesn't know how to take care of his or her hair, your great haircut will quickly look like a disaster. It's not enough to be an excellent haircutter, you also need to teach the do's and don'ts of healthy haircare.

2.1 THE THINGS TO DO

A. **The Rules are Simple.**
Following the do's takes the least possible time, money, concern, and resource use, while it also maximizes the hair's growing health and healthy appearance.

1. Shampoo daily or at least every other day.
This is the first and most important rule for healthy hair. By keeping hair and scalp clean you control dandruff, give the hair a healthy sheen, and the hair is able to maintain a good shape and appearance throughout the day. These benefits are easily achieved with a two or three-minute shampoo and towel-dry.
If the hair is shampooed every-other-day, on the day without a shampoo, wet the hair with warm water, give it a good rub and towel-dry. The "bed-head" problem is no more.

2. Use the hands for a comb.
When you teach people to groom their hair by hand combing, you're helping make life a little easier. No longer will they have to be sure their comb or brush is with them at all times, but more important, the old preoccupation with every hair being in place becomes an unnecessary part of the past. Hand combing is relaxed and extra easy, and your comb is always at your fingertips.

3. Give yourself a scalp massage.
A vigorous massage turns a pale-white scalp to a warm-pink color by increasing blood flow to the top of the head. It's a healthy treat for the follicles, and it feels good too.

4. Get a haircut every month or two.
When those old (perhaps damaged) ends get cut off and you remove hard-to-manage hair length, your efforts are rewarded by hair that is healthy and easily maintained. A precision haircut, cut to the right length and shape, is not only the key to an easy shampoo, it also keeps the hair well shaped after hand combing or a scalp massage.

B. RESISTANCE TO THE DOS.
For many people, simple haircare makes sense--share your knowledge and they get right into it. For many others you can expect opposition to the do's. Change is hard for most folks, and with the above prescriptions you're pushing for significant change.

What you're up against

I hate to shampoo!

There are many reasons why people don't shampoo very often. The more common ones are fear of hair loss and much pain that comes from tangled hair;

It takes too much time!

They need to spend too much time and effort taming the messiness that a shampoo creates.

Hand combing? No way!

The old notion that every hair must stay in "its" place all day long is held by many.

What you can do

I hate to shampoo!

Teach basic hair knowledge such as the stages of hair growth and shedding, and the need to control dandruff. Explain why hair gets snarled and how cutting off those ends makes the difference.

It takes too much time!

Explain how a precision haircut that cuts off excess length gets rid of messy, time-consuming hair. A 2 to 3 minute shampoo and towel-dry is all it takes.

Hand combing? No way!

The big problem here is convincing folks to dump the idea that every hair must be like its cast in bronze. The I-must-be-in-complete-control-at-all-times approach is a frustrating way to handle 100,000 hairs. A windy day won't be a bad day with the hand-combed approach.

There are a number of benefits to those who get the haircuts and adopt the kind of haircare this book recommends. Simple, easy haircare convinces many, but perhaps the biggest bonus comes from replacing the old "every-hair-must-stay-in-its-place" rule with the relaxed approach that makes hand-combing and scalp massage possible. These photos will help convince them--each set of photos show hand combed hair, before and after the haircut.

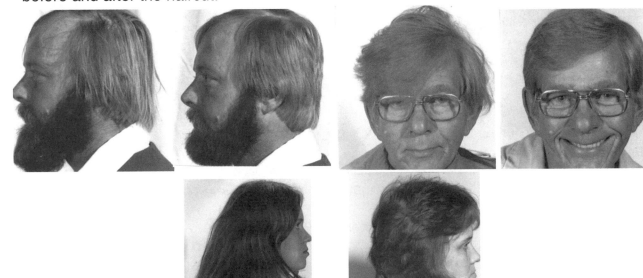

C. How-To For The Do's

1. The right way to shampoo. Shampoo and towel-dry every day, or at least every other day. Most people find the first thing in the morning is the best time to do it because sleeping usually makes messy hair with it being bent and kinked, especially around the sides. Make it the first task of the day and the hair is usually air-dried in less than a half-hour. If the hair is shampooed every other day it should be thoroughly wetted with warm water and towel-dried on the mornings it's not shampooed--this will remove those kinks. The goal whenever you shampoo is to do a thorough cleaning job. Getting the hair really clean means removing all the dirt, dandruff and oils that coat the scalp and hair shafts. When the hair is 100% clean, (one or two shampoo applications usually does it), the hair squeaks as your finger tips grasp and slide out on a group of hair shafts. This is the sound you want to hear on the hair all over the head. Here's how:

a. Pre-scrub. If the hair isn't shampooed daily, spend a minute massaging the scalp to loosen dirt and dandruff. This is best done with a plastic brush with widely spaced bristles (the next chapter shows the right kind).

b. Shampoo application. Wet the hair and scalp with warm water and apply a small amount of shampoo to the hands. You probably won't get much lather on this first shampoo application--you'll get that if a second application is given.

c. Getting it clean. Rub the shampoo between hands and distribute evenly over the outer layer (ends) of the hair. Use a rotary motion to work the shampoo down to the scalp with finger tips or brush. Give the hair and scalp a fairly vigorous workout, but don't be rough with the hair.

d. **Rinse thoroughly**. Poor rinsing leaves a film, preventing the hair from having sheen.

e. Check for squeaks. If you don't hear a squeaking sound as you handle the hair, give one more application of shampoo.

f. Towel-dry. With shorter hair you can do a fairly vigorous towel-drying, but with longer hair, particularly fine hair, you should wrap the towel around the hair and "blot" it dry. Remember, wet hair is prone to breakage in its softened condition--longer, fine hair even more so.

g. Grooming. After the towel-dry, use a brush with widely spaced bristles to gently brush the hair in the direction you want it to lie. The hair lies best if your brushing goes along with the hair's grain, or only slightly bends away from the grain. Let the hair air-dry and follow up with another brushing. If you're in a hurry for the hair to dry after towel drying or you want to impart a little extra fullness to the hair, a blow-dryer can be used or the hair can be "drum-dried" with your fingers (chapter 5 shows how).

2. Shampooing the Little Folks

Many adults **hate** to shampoo--one glance at their hair and it's obvious who they are.. This attitude is a result of what was done (or not done) in their early years. Children, from infancy to age four or five, need special handling if they are to grow up with a positive attitude toward shampooing. All the shampoo how-to rules apply to the little ones, in addition practice:

• **A gentle touch**. In a child's first year, take extra care to avoid putting pressure on the soft spot on the top of the head. Children, up to about school age, are usually quite sensitive to any kind of pressure on their scalp--go slow and easy with them. Youngsters normally have fine hair that likes to tangle--be sure it's thoroughly brushed out before shampooing.

•**The recline way to shampoo**. For a child's first four to five years, the parent should shampoo their hair for them using the recline method of shampooing. Explain to them that this is the same method used in barber and beauty shops: The shampooer lays the head back (face toward the ceiling) into the shampoo bowel. This can be accomplished at home by using a high stool in front of a sink or by cradling them back in a tub. When a child sits up in a tub or stands in a shower, they always end up with water and shampoo getting in their eyes--no wonder so many children grow up hating to shampoo!

• **Use low pH shampoo.** Frequent shampooing requires the use of mild, low pH (also called acid-balanced) shampoos. For children with their finer-textured, more damage-prone hair this prescription is extra important. While some "no-tears" baby shampoos have adopted the low pH approach, some are still strong stuff--they may not sting the eyes, but the hair damage I've seen on tikes who used this stuff, tells me there ought to be a law (it always cleared-up when they switched over to low pH shampoos).

3. How to Hand comb

Simply use your fingers as if they were the teeth of a comb. Exactly which way you do this depends on the type of hair, such as:

• **Straight and wavy hai**r. Use your fingers as you would a comb or a brush. The fingertips, instead of the teeth or bristles, reach all the way down to the scalp as the groomers move through the hair. The fingers travel in any direction you like, but if you go with the hair grain (for the most part), you're assured of hair that lays its best.

With a feather-back hairstyle, the hands go in a front-to-back direction. The results come out like this:

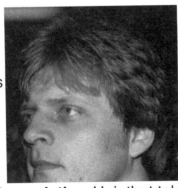

If the top hair wants to go off to one side, a sideways path through the hair gives this appearance:

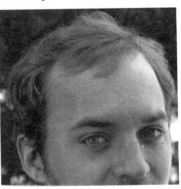

• **The curly and kinky varieties**. Hair that takes a winding path out from the head needs a different approach because it's usually heavy and thick--those blunt fingertips have a hard time moving through the hair.

Use the fingers like a hair pick to make the hair's ends stand out in a smooth shape. To do it, insert your spread-out fingers into the hair and lift out, or grab the hairs between the palm of the hand and the fingertips, then pull straight out. The results come out something like this:

4. The Invigorating Scalp Massage

The objective with a scalp massage is to give some feel-good stimulation, and to promote an extra supply of blood to that pale-white scalp. At the least, an increased flow of blood brings an extra supply of nutrients for the hair follicles, plus it does feel good to move that scalp around.

•The fingertips workout

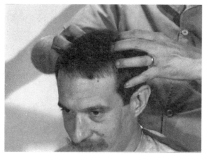

The fingertip pads massage the entire scalp vigorously for a couple of minutes. Use a 2-to-3 inch circular motion with firm downward pressure that moves the scalp. You could also use a massage brush or hair brush in the same way.

This method works well with shorter hair, and with longer hair, if it is undamaged. With damaged hair, you can cause pain. The next approach works best for sick hair.

• The push-it-to-the-top method. Here you use your hands in two different ways:

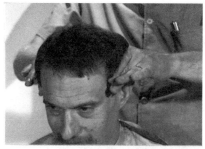
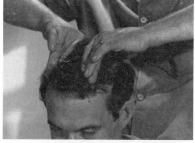

The insides of the hands move from the sides to the top with a firm pressure. Use this same technique with one hand starting at the forehead, and the other at the nape of the neck.

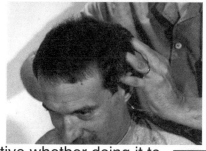
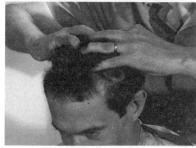

The spread-fingers technique is used in a similar way, but here the fingertip pads are in contact with the scalp.

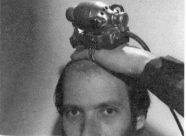

These methods are effective whether doing it to yourself or to someone else. However, if you want to add a whole lot of enjoyment to the massage, use a vibrator massager like the one shown here. If you've never had one of these on your head, you're in for a real treat (great for an aching neck or back too).

2.2 THE HAIR'S GROWING HEALTH AND THINGS TO AVOID

Whether hair keeps growing depends on genetics (no control over that), and what you do or don't do to the hair (quite a bit of control here). Avoiding much in the world of hair products has a big impact on how the hair looks--sick or healthy looking hair is a choice.

1. Crusty scalp. The need for frequent shampooing has already been stressed, but what happens if the scalp is neglected? Follicles, those busy growth factories, like the rest of our outside layer, needs to breathe. An accumulation of dead skin cells (dandruff), sebaceous gland oil, and dirt can produce a covering on the scalp that literally strangles the follicles. This abuse is strictly optional.

2. Hair bending. When you put constant pressure on those delicate hair follicles, you are asking for trouble. Many ponytail wearers have discovered their tightly pulled-back hair has left them with bald patches. This way of wearing the hair is especially damaging to people with a Type 1 hair grain which wants to lie downward on the sides. Pulling the hair back bends the hair near the root, putting more stress on the hair follicles than would occur with a Type 2 hair grain. The technical name for this condition is **traction alopecia**. While usually a temporary hair loss condition, I've seen people with a thinned-out kind of permanent hair loss on the sides.

Another common example of strained follicles occurs with people who bend their top hair, trying to make it lie in a direction that doesn't agree with the hair grain. Straight hair is affected by this, but not wavy and curlier hair--these types can easily lie in different directions when cut short.enough. While stressed follicles on top isn't as severe as it is on a ponytail, I've seen so many people with thinned-out hair where the top hair has been bent for a long time, I have to believe traction alopecia is the culprit. This belief is a result of my 50 years of observations: The more hair bends near the root, the more stress on the follicle; the longer this condition occurs, the greater chance of hair loss. You can fight that hair grain until the hair falls out. On the other hand, you can accept what your genes have given you, and get a precision haircut that results in the hair lying the way it wants. Life with your hair will be much easier, and you'll make the most of your hair's health in the process.

3. Malnutrition of the follicles

When the body is deprived of its basic needs, hair is an early casualty. We start with the crucial one:

a. Protein. If you've ever seen malnourished people you know how important protein is to hair. Without it, you have major hair loss (but who can be concerned about hair when starvation is an everyday concern). Hair loss from this source is usually temporary, but it can become permanent.

b. Minerals. Iron increases the amount of oxygen in the blood, which is important for the growing health of hair. Weak, easy-to-damage hair may reflect a deficiency in zinc, a needed trace mineral.

c. Vitamins. Vitamin E is excellent for the whole circulatory system, so it is important for those follicles and their blood supply. Vitamin C creates a healthy skin and scalp. B vitamins are necessary for normal hair growth.

These essential ingredients to healthy hair can be supplemented in pill form, but the best way is to have a wholesome, well-rounded diet.

2.3 WHAT IT TAKES FOR HEALTHY LOOKING HAIR

Some people have strong hair that flourishes no matter what kind of hurtful things they do to it. Then there are the rest of us who have to take special care to avoid the many ways hair can be damaged. It isn't fair, but...

Before healthy hair is transformed into a pile of straw, it usually goes through a few worsening stages of damage. To begin, you'll notice a lack of sheen--that dullness is caused by the cuticle layer being roughed up instead of lying flat. About this time you get into a somewhat painful brushing or combing stage; instead of moving easily through the hair, the groomer has difficulty, and the follicles let you know pullout pressure is being applied. Then instead of a lack of sheen, the hair now becomes totally drab as it absorbs any light that may hit it. At this point, the hair is entering the frazzled stage with split ends common, and broken hairs showing up in the brush or comb. Now the hair not only makes others wince, it's very painful to attempt any kind of haircare. You get frazzled hair from a variety of causes; however, the worst culprits come from the things we buy. Of course there are beneficial products for hair, but many consumer products must be avoided if we want healthy hair. In the following list, the most common causes of damage come first. Keep in mind that when you have damaged hair, you may have only one cause, but most likely it is caused by some combination of these things.

1. Permanents: Chemical Carnage for Hair

The first don't is the big one. The permanent wave hoax is a multi-<u>billion</u>-dollar-a-year business that causes more damage to human hair than any other single source.
This treatment makes straighter types of hair wavy, curly, even kinky. The hair is rolled up on two-inch long rods, all over the head, and a high-pH chemical solution is applied to alter the way each hair's cells lie alongside each other. After a time, a neutralizer is applied to stop the chemical action of the first application. How curly the hair gets depends on the strength of the chemical solution, and the size of the rods used. Large diameter rods produce a softer, body-wave curl, the smallest rods produce a kinky curl.

Whatever size rods are used, you'll find after the hair has been treated, individual hairs take on the appearance of a stretched-out spring.

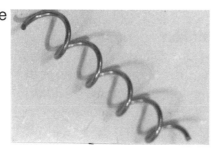

If the hair was given a body-wave perm, the the spring would be stretched out more; a kinky-type perm would be more tightly coiled.

Altering the way hair cells lie alongside each other invites major hair-shaft damage. The outside armor cells normally lie smooth; however, after a perm, they lie rough on the outside of the new curves.

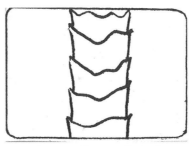
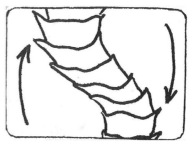

At the very least, a permanent roughs up the cuticle layer, leaving the hair so it's easily tangled and prone to the many ways it can be damaged. At its worst, a perm destroys hair by causing major hair breakage. Between these two extremes, you can expect dull, no-sheen hair, and split ends are also quite common.
Keep these things in mind about permanents:
a. How bad will it be? Permanents have been described as a controlled-damage way to change the natural state of the hair. Being able to "control" this process depends on factors such as the the strength and porosity of the hair, how strong the solution is, how

long it's left on the hair before the neutralizer is applied, and the size of the rods (more damage with smaller diameter rods). These different factors make it difficult to control how much damage is done: It usually takes a few permanents before you can zero-in on the right combination that minimizes damage (but the damage is **only** minimized).

b. The same stuff for a different reason. Hair straighteners are basically the same concoction as permanents, but as the name suggests, it makes the hair straighter. Kinky hair can become curly or wavy, even quite straight; curly and wavy hair can also end up straight or at least lie into soft waves. All the problems associated with permanents are also true for straighteners, but for some reason, hair breakage is much more common.

c. Even the name is a hoax. The dictionary defines permanent as something that is fixed and lasting. Hair permanents are neither of these. The curl hair has right after a perm will slowly return to its natural state; the treated hair may not be totally straight again, but it gets much straighter than right after the perm. Permanents are also temporary because only the treated hair curls--the new growth will be its usual self.

d. The dirty trick about permanents. Perms are usually sold to people with straight, fine, limp hair that lies close to the scalp. The sales pitch promises the hair will have added body and fullness, and it will make shampooing easier. Yes, it does those things, but fine hair is the weakest kind, and it's most prone to the damage of a perm treatment. This book shows how to give straight, small-diameter hair the type of haircuts that maximize the hair's natural body and fullness, and that make wash-and-wear haircare possible. You get all the benefits of a perm without any damage.

Permanents have been around since the 1920s, and they'll probably keep going strong until head-shaving becomes the norm. While most perms are unnecessary, a few people have extra troublesome hair that can benefit from a perm. A perm can be beneficial because when hair is made curly, it stands out from the head. Problem straight hair lies down except for those troublesome areas that like to stand on end. Give it a perm and all the hair stands on end, effectively hiding those problems.

If a perm is given, several things can make matters worse:

•**Avoiding extra damage**. Never give a perm to a head of hair that still has remnants of the last permanent. Get all of the old perm cut off before applying the next chemical blast. When you apply a permanent to hair with old perm on it, you're asking for double or triple damage. This rule applies to hair damaged by other means, such as harsh shampoo or hair coloring. It takes strong, healthy hair to withstand the damage permanents do.

•**Other things to avoid.** Don't use a hair dryer after a shampoo. Always let the hair air-dry after you blot-dry it with a towel. To avoid hair breakage, never brush out the hair while it's still wet. When dry, use a brush with wide-spaced teeth to gently untangle the curls.

2. Strong shampoos.
Coming in a close second behind permanents as the biggest cause of hair damage are the high-pH shampoos available on the retail shelves. Today most shampoos are mild enough for daily use if they list ascorbic acid as one of the ingredients. However, many still wreak havoc:

A. High-pH (alkaline) shampoos. These are mainly old brand-name favorites left over from the 1950s and 60s when most shampooed only once or twice a week. Infrequent shampooing means minimum exposure to the harsh chemicals in these shampoos, and it means you have a large accumulation of natural oil to help protect the hair. These popular shampoos from the past have an alkaline pH level from 7 to 10 or more on the 1 to 14 pH scale; hair and skin is slightly acidic at a 4.5 to 6.0 level.

Since the middle 60s people have developed frequent shampooing habits. Today, a majority prefer the daily "wash and wear" way to care for hair. Many benefits come with the clean hair approach, but if high-pH shampoos are used, hair soon gets to the split ends and breakage stage.

B. Dandruff shampoos. They are getting better, but many of these shampoos are damaging to the hair, if used frequently. People with strong, coarse-textured hair may avoid the damage these shampoos can do, but if it's fine hair, better beware

C. Bar of soap. Some people don't care what they use on their hair, and it shows. Bar soap is usually alkaline, and if used long enough it makes the hair into a frizz-ball disaster. Hair destruction occurs if you're careless when washing the face and neck. Just a little of those soap suds in the hair can result in a split-end disaster on the edges.

3. Hair coloring.

People in the United States spend many BILLIONS a year on coloring their hair. Like permanents, this kind of chemical application is somewhat damaging to hair at best, destructive at worst.

You can tint, frost, foil, streak, rinse, dye, and even bleach those hairs, but when you fiddle with the hair's color, the cuticle layer gets damaged to some degree. It's common to end up with dull hair, split ends, hair breakage, even an inflamed scalp (the worst problems occur when peroxide is used). Studies have indicated some hair-coloring preparations used over many years are the cause of scalp cancer.

4. Electric appliances.

Blow-dryers, curling irons, and other heat-producing gadgets designed to change the appearance of the hair, can turn those poor little hairs into a pile of straw. The change will be gradual, but over time the hair loses its sheen, develops split ends, and can get to the point of breakage.

The haircuts in this book do lend themselves to the use of any type of hair appliance or chemical application, but excellent damage-free results are obtained from the haircare I recommend.

5. Environmental factors.

If you were careful to avoid the above-mentioned causes of hair damage, your hair can still be damaged by things in our environment.

A. The sun. Those solar rays, besides lightening the color of hair (the "summer blond"), also dries out and damages the ends of the hair.

B. Chemicals in water. I am not sure about some of the other chemicals found in water, but chlorine is very hard on hair. I've seen a number of swimmers whose finer-textured hair could not grow long, breaking off before reaching a length of two inches. In extreme cases, I've seen blond hair turn a greenish color.

C. Air. Industrial centers and gas-burning vehicles have combined to make our air unhealthy to those with damage-prone hair. Environmental sources of damage are hard to avoid, but having the hair cut every couple of months removes those overexposed ends before they get to the frazzled stage.

6. Hairsprays and dressings.
These aids do little damage to the hair, but they create a mental strain that serves no worthwhile purpose. It's a losing battle trying to keep those hairs from any kind of movement--a windy day or a little touch can wreck your look and cause distress. Because hairspray floats around the air when used (and gets into lungs etc,) we don't use it in our shop.

7. You have to be an educator.
As with the do's of haircare, the don'ts require changes in habits. Most of us have some difficulty with change, but the haircare changes I recommend are extra hard because of the brainwashing that surrounds hair. To teach about the do's and don'ts of healthy haircare, you must stand up to the massive $ales job the media pushes at us ALL THE TIME. When you consider the average 18-year-old has been bombarded by over a half MILLION television commercials, a mass media outlook on hair and its care is formed at an early age. Added to this is over 40 viewing hours a week; the people seen on T.V. always spend plenty of time with a hairstylist before you see them. The message about how hair's appearance may not be direct, but it is there.

As if media indoctrination weren't enough, plenty of professionals prey on their patron's insecurities and push them into buying all manner of extras that promise "beauty and acceptance." The net result is a lot of people doing foolish, damaging things to their hair, convinced they are doing the right thing.

In the face of all this misinformation, you come along and propose a mostly unknown "natural haircare" approach. When is the last time you heard or saw an ad for natural haircare? This less-is-better way of caring for hair doesn't bring in the big money, but it leaves the hair in the healthiest condition.

Again, it all boils down to you being an educator. After teaching, encourage them to give the simple approach an honest try. They will soon discover what healthy, carefree hair is all about.

2.4 REMEDIES FOR HAIR AND SCALP PROBLEMS

1.Excessive Oiliness
Many people complain about their oily hair, and how it seems worse now than in past years. It's doubtful they're experiencing more sebaceous gland production; instead, they are waking up to the steady flow they've had since puberty. Awareness of oil is tied to the way haircare has changed. In the 1950s and 60s infrequent shampooing was the rule. Men shampooed once a week or less, then smacked their hair down with hairdressing. On average, most women wore their hair longer then, and typically gave it a once-a-week shampoo and set, with much hairspray to hold it till the next week. The longer styles, plus hairspray worn by women, and the greasy stuff men used were effective ways to hide the oil accumulation. With the swing to wash-and-wear haircare, the hair lies fine when it's clean, but when oil gets out on the hair shafts, it makes the

hair lay in strange, contrary ways. The old haircare masked your awareness of the oil; today's haircare lets you know how productive those little glands are.

Some people produce more oil than others, but as noted earlier, there is no way to regulate oil production. You could damage the hair so the cuticle layer cells curl up, thereby slowing the oil's trip to the ends, or.grow the hair long so it takes longer for the oil to reach the ends. However, the only healthy way to control sebum production is by frequent shampooing with mild (low-pH, acid-balanced) shampoo. Most people have to shampoo daily to keep the oil off the hair, however, the haircuts taught here make daily shampooing extra easy, not a chore. Here are a few other things to keep in mind:

• **The right time**. When hair is shampooed has an impact on the oily condition. If you shampoo before bedtime, the oil has an eight-hour head start on the coming day. A morning shampoo prevents the oil showing up on the ends during the middle of the day.

• **What's the source of that odor?** If a person goes several days or more without shampooing, the oil buildup gives off a strong odor. People with this condition don't seem to know how bad that sebum smells. If a customer has this problem, you can convince that person about the need to shampoo more often. Have them wash their hands and smell them; then have them massage their scalp and smell their hands again. The difference in the two smells proves your point, and will encourage frequent shampooing.

• **Strange things happen to hai**r. Whenever hair get loaded with oil, funny-looking things happen:

a.**Wild hair**. Natural oil tends to make a mess of how the hair lies, especially if you have fine-textured hair. The before-and-after shampoo photos below make the point well.

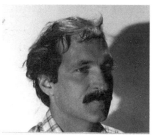 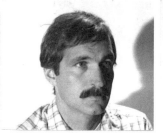 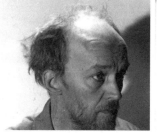 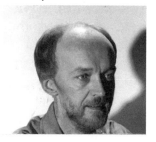

b. A hair-grain clash get worse. A ducktail neckline or a double cowlick has a tendency to stand out from the rest of hair when it's clean, but when the oil builds up you can bet the hair will pop out.

c. The hair type appears to change. Straight hair gets wavy, and wavy hair turns curly. The oil makes the hair stick together, multiplying the hair's tendency to wave or curl.

d. Thinning hair becomes invisible. Oil is heavy enough to make hair lie flat on the scalp, and it makes the hair clump together into strands of many hairs. Those strands have spaces between them which shows off the scalp--a sure way to achieve bare-minimum coverage.

2. **Hair That Doesn't Lie Well**

This common complaint results from a number of different causes. Any of the following can create flippy, messy-lying hair, but when two or more of these conditions are present, things get much worse.

***

The morning is wiser than the evening.   Russian proverb

•**A bad haircut**. Many haircutters either don't know how to give a good haircut, or they just don't care. The precision haircuts you are about to learn solves this problem.

•**Damaged hair**. If the cuticle layer is curled up or the ends are split, the hair lies in all sorts of weird directions, kind of like a pile of straw. Follow the do's and don'ts to a healthy head of hair.

•**Fighting the grain**. When you try to comb or brush straight hair against its natural growth pattern (the hair grain), or if you leave the hair so long that it bends away from its natural lying inclinations, you are guaranteed a head of hair that does not lie well. Cut the hair so it lies the way it wants, and don't force into some contrary position.

•**Thinned-out hair.** Those thinning shears can make a disaster out of any head of hair, especially if they are overused (more on this later in this chapter). Cutting hair with plain haircutting scissors eliminates this source of poor laying hair.

•**Clashing hair grain**. A double cowlick in the crown region or ducktail neckline (especially if you have coarser-textured straight hair) can result in the hair standing out from the head. Solving this problem requires you to get it cut to the right length. (See Chapter 6).

•**Hats.**.I wear a hat when outside to keep from getting a sunburn, and in the winter for warmth. The price I pay for my protection and comfort is messy hair. People with ample hair, who want that hair to lie well, have to avoid wearing hats.

•**Excessive oiliness**. As the last section pointed out, if natural oil coats the hair, the hair clumps together, and usually doesn't lay good. Frequent shampooing is the only answer.

•**Slept-on hair**. It is a rare person who can sleep a night away and not wake up with hair sticking out in different directions. A morning shampoo is the easy remedy.

•**Sweaty hair**. Whenever hair gets sweaty, it lies as it does when excessively oily: When hairs clump together flippy hair results. A shorter haircut during the warmer months helps keep the head cooler.

•**Harsh water**. If the shampoo water has a high mineral content or contains chemicals such as chlorine, your hair may lie poorly. Use rain water or softened water.

The truth is: Hair that lies poorly is optional. Whenever you see it, there's a cause for it and it has a solution. You may have to do a little detective work and spend time educating, but your efforts will be well spent.

3. Static Electricity

If hair stands out from the head when a hat is removed, or the same happens when a comb or brush travels through the hair, static electricity has struck again. This problem only shows itself on straight and wavy hair because this hair normally lies down. Curlier hair types are also affected, but this hair stands out from the head so the effects are hidden. Here is what can be done:

• **Dryness.** Like dandruff, this problem is much worse in the winter when the humidity level is lower, so keep the moisture level higher.

•**Natural versus manmade.** Synthetic fabrics, such as nylon hats. make matters worse than wool or cotton. Hand combing works much better than a plastic comb or brush.

•**A little coating.** A tiny dab of conditioner or lanolin rubbed between the hands and then through the hair usually takes care of it.

***

All that we send into the lives of others comes back into our own.   Edwin Markham

2.5. MENTAL HEALTH BENEFITS

Giving the kind of haircuts taught here has positive and surprising benefits.

•**Carefree hair**. When the haircut allows a person to spend just a couple of minutes a day on their haircare, and then be able to ignore their hair for the rest of the day, no matter what happens to it, that person is more able to partake of life's little joys. People who use spray or hairdressing to keep every hair in place, find these precision haircuts meet their no-change needs perfectly. However, soon they discover their hair stays in a good shape no matter what happens to it--for probably the first time, they have the option of ignoring their hair.

• **A good cut makes you feel better**. A good haircut won't lift a person out of a depression, nor does it transform a negative personality, but it does help to bolster one's outlook. It's hard to pinpoint what it is about a good haircut: For some it's the same feeling you get when you change from grubby clothes. People with sensitive skin like being rid of those bothersome hairs around the ears or neck, and others say it feels good when they move their hands through freshly cut hair. For others it's being able to check a mirror in the morning and like what they see--no more frowns to start the day. Whatever it is, a good haircut makes a positive difference.

• **Less is better**. A person feels good knowing their haircut maximizes the hair's health while it minimizes the amount of resources, time and money spent on the hair. Using minimum resources on hair won't solve environmental problems, but it's good not to add more to the problem than what's absolutely necessary.

•**Spread some quality around.** Whenever a person sees someone at work who knows what to do and how to go about it in the best, most efficient manner, it rubs off on them. It tends to make that person want to do their own work in the best possible way.

All these benefits help to put a little extra bounce in your step.

2.6 THE MYTHS ABOUT HAIR

I doubt there is anything in this world surrounded by more utter nonsense than hair. In my 50 years of haircutting I've heard the full range of tales and legends, quick-fix remedies, and screwball reasons for hair doing what it does. Knowledge of this world of misinformation is important because a large part of what people do--or don't do--to their hair is based on these hair-brained ideas. Our hair mythology begins with the most common one.

A. Hair Fashion

Hair fashions exist, but there's a big myth about being able to adapt to them. We see in the mass-media, or among friends or acquaintances (who have probably been influenced by the media), someone with a becoming hairstyle, and we think that's for me. The problem with this keep-up-with-the-Joneses approach is that rarely will a person who wants a certain look to their hair have the right kind of hair for that look. Hair variables such as the hair-grain, texture, and the type of hair is crucial to the hair's appearance. You can give the best, most appropriate kind of haircut for the look a person has in mind, but if they have the wrong kind of hair, you'll have an unhappy customer on your hands.

A classic example of this folly occurred in the past with "feathered-back" hairstyles. I think these styles, with the sides lying toward the back of the head, and the bangs mostly off the forehead, are a big improvement over the bangs-on-the-forehead styles of the 1960s and 70s. The forehead is oily enough without any help from hair lying on it--a good way to promote acne problems.

Despite the advantages, problems exist when you strive for this kind of haircut. It works great if you have a fairly thick head of hair, and it's slightly wavy with a Type 2 hair grain. For those of us with a Type 1 hair grain, our hair needs bending devices and/or a body-wave permanent to achieve what others manage without much effort.

The endless parade of new hairstyles in the past 20 to 30 years has added momentum to the hair fashion myth. The "latest thing" is created by stylists with money backing of corporations who sell hair products. If it catches on with enough people it can be a huge moneymaker for the corporate backers. Many, if not most, of those who seek these creations are the trendy people who are easily bored (a kind of depression). and who want quick "fixes" for their ego problems.

For the average person, playing the hair fashion game is a losing game. Occasionally they can conform to the latest; most of the time they end up with a style not suited to their hair--unless you get into expensive and damaging ways of changing the natural state of the hair. Large amounts of money, frustration and concern is expended in a game where the rules keep changing (so you're never quite good enough), and damaged hair is the usual outcome. Many have played this no-win game so long, they don't know what it is to have a healthy head of hair

B. Training Hair

The myth that hair will do whatever we want must be laid to rest. Wishful thinking has it that by continuously combing and brushing the hair in the direction you want it to lie, you eventually change the hair's preferred way of lying. As already noted, the grain of the hair is completely unchangeable: When you "train" hair, you simply grow it long enough so it bends into your idea of how it should lie. This is a problem that grows on you: Longer hair is heavy hair, longer heavy hair is a mop that wants to flop around. To keep that hair under control, you must use hairspray or hairdressing, and also keep combing it and combing it. To top it off, those bent hairs are happy to fall out before their time (traction alopecia wins again)

A common example of this myth has to do with the American male, and the left-side part. For unknown reasons, perhaps ignorance about hair grain, it became the custom for males to part their hair on the left side of the head, with the top hair combed over toward the right side, and the rear portion of the top hair combed back over the cowlick region and down the back of the head. If you have straighter hair, this works well only if the hair grain goes that way. If the grain dictates a right side part with the hair growing out toward the left side of the top, a lifelong battle ensues. The hair and a bit of mental health is the loser in this struggle. Chapter 5 shows how to part hair.

Another example of trying to "train" hair occurs with men who try to comb all of the top and upper sides straight back. This kind of haircut, called a pompadour or comb-back, became popular decades ago, but you must have wavy or short curly hair if the top is to easily lie toward the back. Straight hair combs back on top only if it's quite long (three inches or more) so it can bend back away from its forward, natural-lying preferences.

With straight hair, the comb-it-back training battle begins with the kind of stand up problems that occur when the hair is combed against the grain. In time the hair gets long enough to bend back and lie down, but by then you have a heavy mop of hair that's always a struggle to keep in place, especially when freshly shampooed. Besides a messy head of hair, the top is full of bent hairs and stressed follicles.

C. Hair Grows Faster In Some Areas Of The Head

Scalp hairs in the anagen stage are all growing out at the same rate. This uniform growth rate may include a few hairs growing a tad slower or faster than the rest, but this tiny difference can't be seen. The popularity of this myth comes from a few sources:

•Assume you've given an excellent haircut to a person with a Type-2 hair grain. As the hair grows longer, they find the hair stands out from the head around the bottom of the sides. This flippy hair is caused by excess length and the extra weight causing the hair to bend downward from the forces of gravity, rather than lying with the grain toward the back of the head. Whenever hair doesn't lie the way it wants, flippy standout hair results. The uninformed person sees that flipping-out hair, and thinks it grows faster than the rest of the hair.

•With the ducktail neck hair that's common with a type-2 grain, there's often a "hair-grain clash" where the upward grain at the bottom neck hair meets the downward grain higher up on the back of the head. This condition causes some of the back hair back to stand out from the rest of the hair. Those unruly, flippy hairs **appear** to grow faster, but things aren't always as they appear.

• Uneven cutting is another possible cause for this misconception. When the hair is not cut smoothly, the longer hairs tend to stand out as they grow longer (especially noticeable after a shampoo). Again, hairs that stick out from the bulk of the hairs are seen as faster growing hair, but if those hairs were cut right they wouldn't be seen.

D. Cutting Causes Hair to Become Coarser and Grow Faster

Men in particular love this common belief. We tend to think this way because of changes in male beard growth. When we are young, the beard starts as fine, soft hair (peach fuzz), and through time and the action of our hormones, it becomes coarse, fast-growing hair. Because that facial hair is shaved many times during this process of the change, we assume shaving causes that change. Not true. Facial hair gets a coarser texture and grows faster regardless of shaving--changes in hormones during puberty controls the process. *Cutting hair does nothing to the hair other than make it shorter.* The most common example of this hair myth comes up with excessive eyebrow growth common for males over age thirty. Many men avoid cutting those long hairs because they think cutting causes those hairs to grow faster, to become more numerous and coarser. Incorrect! Hormones change short-growing hair into long-growing hair. Nothing you can or cannot do changes this fact of middle age.

The same cutting-causes-faster-growth notion spills over to the hair on our heads, although here an extra factor contributes to this myth. Yes, hair seems to grow faster after a haircut, but it's really a matter of how hair growth shows itself on different hair lengths. If your hair is 5 to 6 inches long, you'll be less aware of your hair's steady growth rate than if your hair is cut to a length of 1 to 2 inches. The shorter a person wears their hair, the more they're aware of the growth rate.

E. Straight Hair Grows Faster Than Curly Hair

There is no significant difference in the growth rate among the different types of hair; however, straight hair does show its growth more. This is due to the way straight hair's ends grow straight away from the follicle and scalp. Curly hair, on the other hand, takes a winding path as it grows, and this hides the actual growth rate.

If a curly-haired person and someone with straight hair both get the same short haircuts at the same time; after a few months of growth their hair is about 1 1/2 inches long. The first illustration shows the visual difference in growth-- the last drawing shows the difference when the hairs are stretched out.

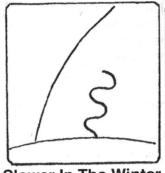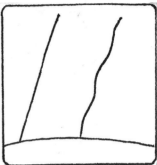

F. Hair Grows Faster In The Summer, Slower In The Winter

Many people are absolutely positive their hair grows faster in the summer, and slower during the cold months. They're a little fuzzy on their reasons, but they stubbornly hang onto this notion. The fact is, growth rate is as steady as the march of time, and neither the temperature nor season of the year has any impact.

One possible explanation for this myth has to do with a fact of haircutting in my home state of Minnesota, U.S.A. Up in this part of the world many, if not most, people tend to grow their hair longer during the cold wind chill months, and wear it on the short side during the warm part of the year. In the winter you have a warm, comfortable ally on your head; during the hot weather your hair is a sweaty burden. If you feel comfortable with your longer hair, you're less likely to be aware of its growth than when it is shorter (and has to be kept short for comfort's sake). With shorter hair in the summer more common, we get back to a question of awareness: Would you be more aware of your monthly 1/2 inch growth if your hair is cut to a length of 1 to 2 inches, or would you notice it more if it's several inches long?

G. Too Much Shampooing Causes Baldness

Wrong! Wrong!! Wrong!!! When you shampoo, you unavoidably remove a large portion of the 100 or so hairs you are bound to shed each day. Those telogen-stage hairs accumulate at the bottom of the sink, and it looks like another big step toward a shiny scalp. (A bigger pile of hair is seen if you don't shampoo often). If you hadn't shampooed, that hair would have been lost in less observable ways--as you brushed or combed, or as a new hair growing beneath the old one pushed it out. You have a much better chance to keep your hair growing if you keep the hair and scalp clean.

H. Shampooing Makes The Hair Less Manageable

Natural oil, hairdressing or hairspray, have enough weight and sticking power to keep hair held down. Shampooing removes these "restraints", and the hair is free to lie in whatever direction it wants. Two conditions don't get along with hair being free to lie the way it wants. These conditions affect any head of hair, but straighter hair has the most problems.

1. Botched haircut. When hair is unevenly cut, it must have the extra weight of natural oils, hairdressing or hairspray to smack it down and keep the hair from showing its poor cutting. This situation was common in the early years of my career when precision haircutting was rare and poor haircuts were the rule--extensive use of thinning shears was largely to blame. Heavy-duty hairdressing (greasy kid's stuff) was necessity to keep hair from looking scary.

2. Fighting the hair grain. When a person is unaware of, or doesn't respect the natural lying preferences of their hair, heavy holding help is needed to coax those stubborn hairs into that person's dreams and schemes.

When either a bad haircut or fighting the grain (or both) of these conditions exist, shampooing does make hair less manageable. A person with these conditions usually has to wait 1 to 3 days after shampooing before their hair doesn't produce a scare when a mirror is seen (more time is needed if no hairdressing or spray is used). Because both hair grain battles and chopped-up haircuts are **optional,** this notion of unmanageability from shampooing is another myth.

The precision haircuts you're about to learn makes shampooing a simple part of daily living, instead of a time-consuming chore. All that's needed is a little acceptance of the hair's natural lying preferences, and unmanageable hair becomes a thing of the past.

I. Different Shampoos Are Necessary for Oily, Normal, or Dry Hair

I suggest you avoid brands of shampoo that have a "oily,"" normal," and "dry hair" version. I've used Nitrazine paper to test the differences between the three versions: I've found shampoos for oily hair usually have a higher pH than dry-hair shampoo. High pH (high alkaline) shampoos are strong concoctions that, over time, cause severe hair-shaft damage.

Perhaps the reason different versions of the the same shampoo came into being has to do with a strong shampoo's ability to produce abundant lather, making it extra effective in removing oil from the hair.

Another possibility is a strong shampoo's ability to create a roughed-up cuticle layer. This effectively slows the oil's trip to the ends of the hair shafts, where it's most noticeable. It's pretty obvious which of these two hairs would slow down the oil:

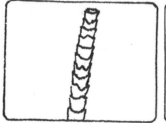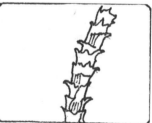

No shampoo made has any impact on the amount of sebum produced by those sebaceous glands--the aging process, hormones and genetics takes care of the oil quantity. Most people have to shampoo daily to keep natural oil under control, and shampooing this often without damaging the hair requires the use of a low pH shampoo.

J. Growing Hair Long to Cover Up Thinning Hair

Men cling to this one; even some women who find their hair thinning in later life think this is the only way to go. Wrong again. Because of the extra weight, long hair lies flat on top of the head, reducing the hair's natural fullness. When you add to that the excess oils or hairdressing and spray needed to keep those longer hairs from flopping around, the result is starkly thin-looking hair.

Hair in this condition sticks together in strands of 10 to 100 hairs, revealing a shiny scalp underneath. Which do you think gives better coverage:

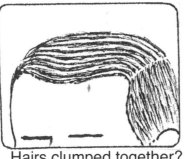 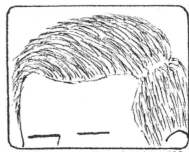

Hairs clumped together?   Each standing by itself?

The best way to handle thinning hair is to cut it on the short side (usually 1 1/2 to 2 inches depending on the fineness or coarseness of the hair). Then, with a shampoo at least every other day, the hair has body and appears more full because the hairs don't stick together in strands of 10 to 15 hairs..The clean-hair approach makes the most of what you have, while providing maximum growing health to the survivors. An added bonus comes on windy days--it's always a bad day for those who wear a "flap", but a short cutting can go through a hurricane without looking scary.

K. Men and Women Need Different Hair Products
Yes, there are differences between the sexes and their hair. The balding or thinning process affects men much more than women. Some men experience a short-growing hair problem around the bottom edges of their head of hair; a problem not found on women. Despite these minor exceptions, no real difference exists between the two sexes in terms of their hair, and they do not require different procedures or products to keep their hair healthy. As fas as I can tell, hair products labelled for men or women are just Madison Avenue hype.

L. Permanents Create Carefree Hair
Billions of dollars are spent annually by people who are told, "If you want shampoo and towel-dry hair, and be able to forget it for the rest of the day, you need a permanent". Another favorite sales approach is built around the permanent's ability to give limp hair some extra fullness, also called "volume" by the sellers.
The kind of haircuts you learn here proves you don't need a permanent to have low-maintenance hair, and you can get maximum fullness without the expensive treatment. If you want to change your natural hair into something wavy, curly or kinky, a permanent is the answer, but you pay much more than money for that change.

M. Thinning Shears Are the Tool to Use On Thick, Heavy Hair
No, in fact, the over use of thinning shears is one of the worst things that can be done to any head of hair. Typically the cuts start at about the halfway point on the hair shafts that your hand (or comb) is holding. Those toothed cutters take one "chomp" there, and perhaps another cut closer to the ends as the hand slides further out on the hair shafts. Thinning is usually done to the top hair, but sometimes it's done all over the head. The net result is some of the hairs get cut short, some are cut a little longer, and many are left uncut.

***

It's good when our hair doesn't cause others to feel sympathy or concern.   Anonymous

If you do this to any type hair, especially coarse hair, you get a lot of shorter hairs standing straight on end, and pushing out neighboring, longer hairs.

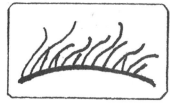 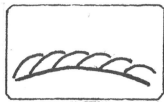

Thinned-out hair   No thinning

Thinning shears also result in poor lying hair because they make partial cuts on the hair. To explain this, we need to take a close look at what happens when the blade with 28 to as many as 46 teeth meets the cutting blade.

Many hairs are held by each small indentation on the top of the teeth--these are the hairs that get cut.

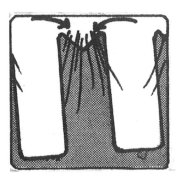 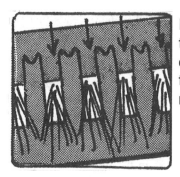

However, most of the hair slips down between the teeth, and remains uncut.

When the cutting blade closes down on the teeth, each indentation holds too much hair. Most hairs get cut, but some get squeezed off to the edge of the indentation where the hair is partially cut. The thinners nick the hair shafts, and the result looks like stomped-on straw.

Hair damaged by the use of thinning shears.

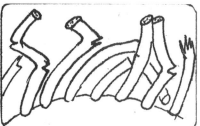 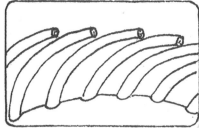

Hair cut by plain scissors.

When you combine the above illustration with a lot of short hairs pushing out longer hairs, you have a hairy disaster. Besides looking scary, this method of dealing with thick hair results in damaged hair and poor haircare:
• **The wounded-armor layer**. When a hair shaft is nicked, the soft cortex layer is exposed, making the hair very prone to damage such as split ends and breakage.
•**Oh no, not a shampoo!** Those who've had their hair thinned-out have an awful time with clean hair because shampooing removes the heavy natural oil (or whatever else holds it down), freeing those nicked hairs to stand out in all directions. If a shampoo produces scary-looking hair, you'll avoid it and probably end up with a cruddy scalp.

The best way to handle thick, heavy hair is to cut it as short as possible, particularly on top, with plain scissors. When you cut off the excess length while leaving the hair just long enough to lie well, you have effectively thinned out the hair without doing any damage. I use thinning shears on a couple of my curly-haired customers: Their hair seems to lay a little better with a limited thinning (one cut out near the ends on each handful of hairs). Also, I use them sparingly on a couple of customers with problem hair.

N. Razor-Cutting Is the Best Way to Cut Hair So it Lies Well

The notion that a better haircut results when you slice the hair with a razor sounds plausible. Advocates say a razor cut leaves each hair's ends slightly tapered so all the ends lie extra smooth. If fact, you create two hair problems with the sliced approach, and precision haircutting is virtually impossible using a razor.

• **Slicing the ends of the hair**. This kind of cutting leaves the cortex layer of the hair much more exposed than it is when cut by scissors. With the soft cortex exposed, the hair is extra vulnerable to being damaged.

• **Curled-up ends**. Razor-cutting results in hair ends that curl up; a close view of hair cut this way reveals a head full of frizzy ends that stand out from the rest of the hair.

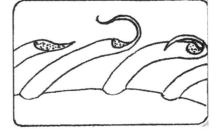

•**Don't move.** Success with razor-cutting requires the customer to hold very still, and the haircutter needs the exact same pushing pressure of the cutting blade against the hair ends. With experience, you may be able to do a good cutting job; however, then you still have the unhealthy consequences shown above.

As in the use of thinning shears, this is an imprecise way to cut hair that leaves hair sick or, at least, in a damage-prone condition. This book teaches how to pull the hair out from the scalp and cut it so it inflicts the least possible damage on the inner layers. The blunt cut with scissors is, by far, the healthiest method of cutting hair.

O. If You're Born Without Hair, You'll Go Bald Early

According to this myth: If you're born with abundant hair, you won't go bald; if you come into the world with a hairless scalp, you have no hope of keeping the hairs that eventually do appear. What will they think of next?

While many bald men have been born with a shiny scalp, and there are many men who kept a full head of hair, who happened to be born with abundant hair, it's also true that the opposite conditions occur with equal frequency.

I find it interesting that hair has mysteries surrounding it, (even dermatologists don't have all the answers on baldness), but this is a very feeble attempt to explain baldness.

P. Wash-and-Wear Haircare Requires Too Much Work

Yes, a shampoo and towel-dry every day or two is too much toil if the hair is poorly cut, or the hair is extra long, or the hair must bend to lie in a direction that's against the grain. These situations make the clean hair approach a drudgery not worth the effort.

No, wash-and-wear haircare is not too much work if the hair is given the precision haircuts taught here, and you accept the natural lie of your hair. In fact, a haircut every couple of months and a 2 to 3 minute shampoo and towel-dry every day or two takes much less time than any other approach: The haircut ensures your hair won't need attention during the day. That amounts to a few minutes out of a day's 1,440 minutes: 3/1440 of a day to make those hairs ignorable and as healthy as can be.

Q. Hair Keeps Growing After You Are Long Gone

Yes, there's even a fairly popular myth about hair and death. This legend has it that a person's hair continues growing after they've died. No. When your physical plant stops operating, the growth factories also quit. Hair does appear to grow after death because of a limitation in measuring hair's growth. You measure a hair from the skin or scalp to the hair tip. Yes, a few days after death, longer hair will protrude from the skin or scalp, but this is a consequence of human physiology. Our bodies are made up of over 90 percent water. When we die, we start dehydrating; that is, we shrink and shrivel because the body's water evaporates. Hair, in contrast, is composed of lifeless cells that don't have any significant moisture content, thus It does not shrink. As the skin surrounding the hair shaft (the root and the bulb) shrinks inward, the hair remains constant, adding a little more distance between the skin and the hair tip. It's the illusion of hair growth, not the reality.

R. You Need Innate Creative Talents To Be a Skilled Haircutter

This common myth is promoted by professional haircutters. The ordinary person watching the haircut process doesn't see much rhyme or reason to what is going on: A snip here and a snip there, throw in a little fancy tool handling, add a dash of double-talk, show them some decent results while gently extolling your "magic", and you have them hoodwinked into thinking this haircutting business is beyond an ordinary person's abilities. This mystification of the craft is understandable from the point of view of wanting to preserve one's livelihood, but understandable or not, it's still a myth. Haircutting is very teachable. As you read on and put into practice this book's how-to, you'll see that haircutting requires no special abilities. You, like millions before you, can learn how to give excellent, precision haircuts.

Hair myths have come about because of the many mysteries surrounding those little thread-like things that grow from our bodies. The uninformed try to make sense of it, and myths come into being. These are the more common ones, and enough is enough. Our next, more positive subject, gets us into haircutting.

***

Everyone does better when everyone does better.

Bumper sticker

Shared joy is double joy. Shared sorrow is half sorrow.

Swedish proverb

Those who make peaceful revolution impossible will make violent revolution inevitable.

John Fitzgerald Kennedy

Plutocracy makes democracy impossible.

Anonymous

Question authority!

Bumper sticker

Question the answers!

Bumper sticker

CHAPTER 3 HAIRCUTTING OVERVIEW

3.1 THE HAIRCUT CURRICULUM

You will learn to give four basic haircuts. The first three are called "Layered Cuts" and the last is a perimeter or "One-Length Cuts" To fill out your bag of skills, you'll be taught several shaping variations for each of these primary ways to cut hair. You begin with one of the easiest and most popular haircuts.

A.The Equal-Length Haircut. There are several names for this excellent haircut such as the "Same-length Cut", the "90 Degree Cut" and more. Whatever the name, the cutting methods used on this haircut are also used on many other kinds of haircuts.

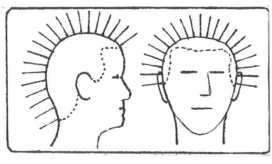 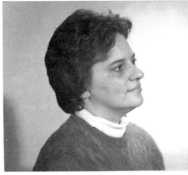 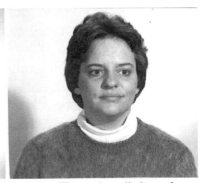

If ever the notion of "beauty in simplicity" applied to a haircut, this is it. The simplicity of this cut is probably why it's been--and continues to be--one of the most popular ways of wearing one's hair.

B.The Long, Layered Haircut. This is the second haircut in your sequence of learning. I suggest holding off on giving this cut until you've mastered the first one. The longer hair is harder to handle and this cut has some advanced tool handling. This haircut goes by different names: "The Long Shag Cut" and the "180 Degree" are a couple of them.

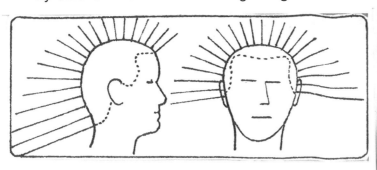 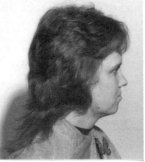 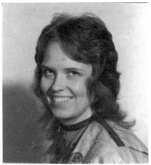

C. The Short, Full Haircut. This is a longer (more full) version of a short haircut. The short length and the tapering involved in this haircut makes it the most difficult of the three layered haircuts. By the time you're comfortable with the first two cuts, you'll be in good shape to handle this one.

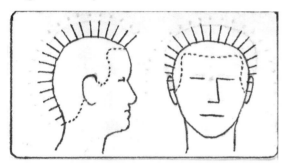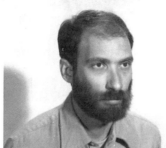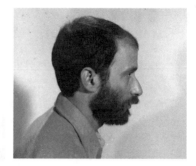

D. The "Bob" Cut. This haircut has been popular since the 1920s. The popularity comes from a longer hair appearance that is cut quite short--some of this and some of that. Unlike the previous haircuts, this cutting is done with the hair lying close to the scalp and skin.

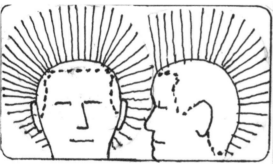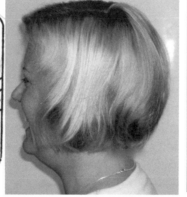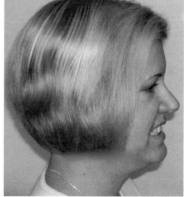

3.2 YOU NEED A SYSTEM

You may have watched a professional cut hair with a "here a snip, there a snip" approach. They cut all around the head several times without a pattern to their cutting. Good haircuts sometimes result from this helter-skelter approach, but it takes years of haircutting experience to make it happen. As a beginning haircutter you need a step-by-step, definite system to the way you cut hair. Skim through any of the haircut chapters to see the systematic way every hair gets cut.

3.3 THE HAIRCUT PROCEDURE IN A NUTSHELL

The first three basic haircuts has you pull the hair out from its normal lying position, hold it in a "standout" position and cut off a predetermined amount of hair. The fourth haircut gets a different treatment with the hair cut while in a lie-down position. All the haircuts follow a step-by-step sequence of cuts, moving in a definite pattern on the head of hair. Your hands and tools assume some different positions in different parts of the haircut and there are minor differences in how you handle the tools with each of the haircuts.

3.4 HAIR THAT LIES LIKE SHINGLES-ON-A-ROOF

The first day I went to barber school in 1963, my Dad, who has been a barber since the I920s, gave me these words of haircutting wisdom: "Always remember, when you cut hair evenly it will lay like shingles-on-a-roof". His advice applied to haircuts that has you hold the hair out from the scalp with your hand or a comb as you do the cutting (the first three haircuts you'll learn). Dad was primarily concerned with the shorter clipper haircuts popular then, but his shingles analogy also produces the best possible results with longer scissor-cut styles.

To portray this shingles notion, assume you're giving a haircut to someone with straight or wavy hair. Once a handful of I,000 hairs (give or take a hundred or two) are cut, and the holding hand releases them, the cut hairs bend back into a lying position. The last illustration in this set magnifies the hair's ends so the shingles idea shows.

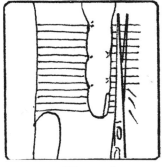

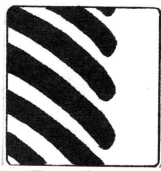

The ends of the hair lie like carefully positioned shingles.

| The cut | The bent lie | The ends |

The first illustration shows the hair being cut so each hair has the same length--the way it's done with an equal-length haircut. A long, layered cut has a gradually increasing length around the sides and back. The shingles principle still holds, but here the hair ends lie farther from each other than they do with the equal-length cut.

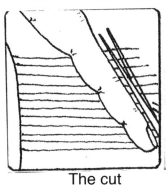
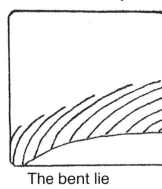
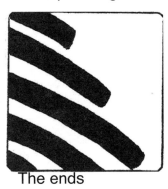

More distance between the edges of the "shingles" when given this kind of cutting.

| The cut | The bent lie | The ends |

***

Nobody can be perfect unless he admits his faults, but if he has faults how can he be perfect?

Lawrence J. Peter

He who cannot forgive others breaks the bridge over which he himself must pass.

Confucius

Never go to a doctor whose office plants have died.

Erma Brombeck

A short, full haircut's decreasing length on the sides and back places the ends a little closer than it is with an equal-length cut.

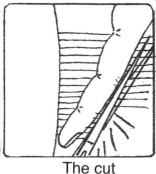 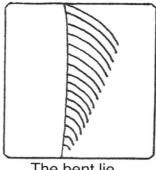 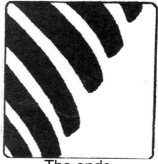

Less distance between those "shingles" with this way of cutting.

The cut   The bent lie   The ends

When hair is cut to lie like shingles, those hairs are able to lie in any direction and they still keep their shingles nature. The fact that those hair ends always blend with their neighbors is the thing that makes these *basic* haircuts so carefree--be it windblown, hand combed, or whatever, it still lies like perfectly placed shingles on a roof.

Thus far the shingles-on-a-roof comparison has shown single cuts for each of the three layered haircuts. However, a haircut consists of many cuts--if you are not consistent in the length you leave the hair, from one cut to the next, you'll have a very poor haircut. The goal with any of the haircuts is to have each cut you make blend with the neighboring cuts. This goal is achieved by following the sequence of cuts and pathways each haircut has, and by using the guide-hair aid (explained later). Doing the practice exercises (found in chapters 4 and 5) builds the hand skills needed to realize the goal of smooth, precision haircuts.

The precision haircutting you learn in this book not only makes hair lie like "shingles", it is the **KEY** to the kind of simple natural haircare described in the previous chapter. When hair is given a precision cutting with the excess length cut off, a shampoo and towel-dry every day or two is not a chore, it's great way to start the day. A few minutes spent on easy haircare makes the hair and scalp as **healthy** as possible, and it keeps the hair **looking good** throughout the day

3.5 THE CUTTING LINE

The main part of a haircut is called bulk-cutting or bulk-removal. The numerous cuts made during this part of the haircut will shorten every hair on the head. As you go through a head of hair making these cuts, one hand holds the hair out from the head while the other does the cutting. The hair is held between two fingers, and they are positioned just below an imaginary line, called the cutting line. After the held hair is cut, the freshly cut ends will touch this cutting line while the hair is still in its stand out from the head position.

This cutting line idea is included here so you'll know the overall goal of all the cuts you make during the bulk-cutting part of the haircut. The heavy line in these illustrations is the cutting line you strive for, as the hair is held out from the head for each cut made during the bulk-cutting. The little marks outside the cutting line represent the hair that has been cut.

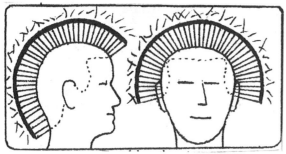

Equal-length cut

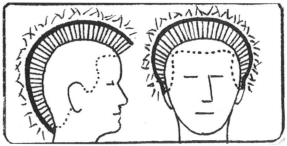

Short, full cut

These two haircuts have you pulling the hair straight out from the scalp, all over the head of hair while doing the bulk-cutting.

To get increasing length around the sides and back of the long, layered cut, the top hair is cut with the hair held straight up from the head. Then the side and back hair is pulled up and cut off, while you maintain the same cutting line that was used for the top hair. Overall you have this cutting line.

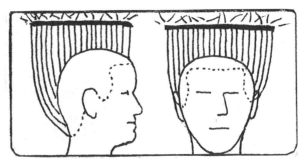

Long, layered cut

Cutting the Bob has your focus on the cutting line shown here:

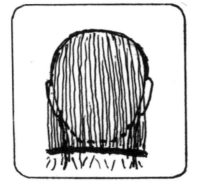

This versatile haircut has several variations that are also explained, however the basic cutting line shown here is used.

3.6 PREPARATIONS FOR HAIRCUTTING SUCCESS

I'm always looking for ways to make my work a little easier or more efficient, but some things can't be avoided. That's the way it is with these preliminaries: they're all necessary to get people-pleasing results on your first haircut.

• Read through the chapters I through 7 as many times as necessary to get a full understanding of what you want to do and how you'll go about doing it.

• Take care in whom you choose for your beginning haircuts. The last chapter's sections on "Cutting Children's Hair" and "Haircutter as Merchant of Change" are helpful in choosing the right ones to begin your haircutting.

• Using the information in chapter 6, analyze your patron's hair and decide the best length and shape for the hair. Communicate your analysis and reach an agreement on what is to be done.

• Once you know what length is intended for your haircut, do the practice exercises: they help get you comfortable with the hand-tool manipulations used during the haircut.
• Heed all the safety considerations that haircutting requires (see subject index for a review before you begin).
• Set up the best possible working environment. Good lighting and tools, adequate rest and no distractions makes it much easier.
• If possible, shampoo and dry the hair before starting. Squeaky-clean hair is a big help.

3.7 THE STEPS

To cut 100,000 hairs with maximum success, the beginning haircutter usually needs to go through seven to as many as nine steps in the haircut procedure. Some heads of hair won't need all the steps, and with experience some may be unnecessary. Assuming you're a beginner and your customer needs all of these steps, this is how you'll do it.

1.Wet the hair. Use a spray bottle to thoroughly wet the hair. Scissor cutting always works better on wet hair. Expect to wet it again during the haircut.
2. Approximate cutting. This step and the next one may not be necessary if you're cutting off less than two inches. If your cutting removes more than 2 to 3 inches, cut an edge-line around the perimeter of the hair. This preliminary cutting is done the same as the final edging, but here the hair is left at least an inch longer than what is wanted for the final laying length.
3. More approximate cuts. This step, like the last one, makes your bulk-removal efforts easier if you will be cutting off more than a couple of inches. Pull out and cut off the excess hair length in 10 to 15 places all over the head of hair. Again, leave the hair at least an inch longer than what you want for the final length. Both the second and third steps make the next step easier to do.
4. Bulk-cutting. This part of the haircut takes the biggest portion of your time and efforts. Despite the time spent here, the cut-by-cut instruction makes this cutting easy to do. With the bulk-removal cuts made here, the main skill to develop is the ability to hold the hair out from the head with the correct holding-hand position. The aids you'll learn make bulk-removal cutting easy to learn.
5. Check for uniform length. Experience eliminates this step, but as a beginner it's an important step. This is done by pulling hair strands straight out from the scalp in a number of locations and measuring their length with a ruler. Length differences of more than a half inch require re-cutting now.
6. Second-time-through. For the beginner, this smooth-off part of the haircut makes the difference between an excellent haircut and a good one, (with experience you probably won't need to do this). You go over the hair you cut during the bulk-removal, but now the holding-hand is held in a different way so you can see and cut any minor length variations. The hair you cut may not fill a thimble, but that's usually enough.
7. Final edging. This finishing step has you cut the edge hairs all around the head. The rule is: cut off very little hair. The bulk-removal cutting has already cut the edge hair.
8. Extra hairs. Most mature males need their nose, ears, and eyebrow hairs trimmed. Males and females need the stray neck hairs trimmed.

9. Last-minute look-over. You may have to do some last-minute cutting to achieve your best results. With the hair dried and brushed out, give it a good inspection and make any necessary corrections.

10. After the Haircut Brush the hair and let them see how well the "shingles" are lying on the roof. Show them what happens with a hand combing--now they'll know what a positive difference comes from a precision cutting. It's not enough to give excellent haircuts, you also have to teach the do's and don'ts of healthy haircare. Share your knowledge--the results are always positive.

Whether your haircut needs all the steps, or some lesser number, this way of going about it gets the job done right

3.8 YOUR TOOLS

Giving precision haircuts requires quality tools that effectively do the task you want them to do. The comb(s) has to easily handle the hair, and allow you to manipulate the scissors in the best possible way. The scissors must be able to cut all the hair you want to get cut--not with two or three or five opening and closing of the cutter, but with just one snip. You need a brush with wide-spaced teeth, one that's able to thoroughly brush the hair by getting all the way down to the scalp.

You can spend $1,000 for a pair of scissors-- 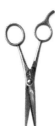 my $50 cutters does the job very well.

These 3 combs and brush cost a total of $10. I also have white combs-- using black combs on light hair and white ones on dark hair helps to see the hair better when I'm using clipper over comb.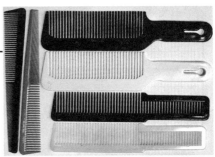

I show how to use a clipper to finish off the bottom neck hair on two haircuts in the book. The clipper here is extra close cutting, and does a good job on edge hairs; the larger one plus an attachment is good at getting the beard cut to the right length. Cost is $100+ for both.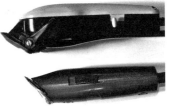

If you want to make a fun career of it and have your own business, add the cost of a good serviceable barber chair and backbar, clippers and sanitizing equipment, a barber pole and miscellaneous odds and ends--all can be bought for less than two thousand dollars. Add the cost of barber school and licensing, which varies from state to state. I don't know of any other professions that can be set-up so inexpensively.

***

Be pleasant until 10:00 in the morning and the rest of the day will take care of itself.

Elbert Hubbard

Mean people breed little mean people.

Bumper sticker

A study of police records shows that a woman has never shot her husband while he was doing dishes.

Anonymous

CHAPTER 4 BULK-CUTTING

4.1 THE "KNACK" FOR USING TOOLS

Many people believe you have to be born with a special ability, called a "knack," to handle tools with ease. I don't agree. To me, this is a tired old excuse for staying in the safety of a narrow rut, for not trying something new.

No, you don't need a "knack" to make things by hand. You can get comfortable with hand-tool activities, but, you must:
• Be clearly taught the correct, most efficient way to handle tools.
• Give yourself enough time to gradually improve skills as you gain experience. You have to be a little patient with yourself during the process.

The first ingredient is my responsibility; the second is yours. Like all beginners, you'll go through a "rookie" stage where your movements are slow and deliberate, and you feel uncomfortable and awkward. Be assured, in a short time tool handling will be second nature to you. It feels comfortable and you won't have to think about each little movement of the tools and hands.

4.2 THE BULK-CUTTING PART OF THE HAIRCUT

Bulk-cutting, also called bulk-removal, is the process of cutting the heavy, hang-down hair that tangles and musses so easily. This kind of cutting is what is used on layered haircuts--it takes the majority of your time as you repeat one basic tool-handling procedure many times all over the head of hair. The same, but slightly different, hand-tool manipulation is used if you do the second-time-through cutting. Bulk-removal cutting consists of combing the hair out from its lying position; grasping the hair with the left hand between the two holding fingers; positioning the two "spacer" fingers so the right length is set up; and cutting the hair that protrudes above the hand. This chapter teaches how to do the bulk-removal for the equal-length haircut. The slightly different bulk-cutting techniques for the two advanced layered haircuts are explained in those haircut chapters.

4.3 POSITIONING TOOLS IN THE TOOL HAND

Before you can use your tools you have to know how to hold them. (It's easier to follow these directions if scissors and comb are in hand.)

A. Beginning Position of the Scissors.
In this position the scissors can be tucked away so the comb can also be used by the tool hand--a busy hand, but not too busy.
• Place your ring finger in the finger grip, between the first and second joints. Bend the finger at both joints. (The "first joint" is the first one from the finger's tip.)
• Place your slightly bent little finger on the tang, near the first joint.

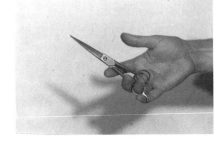

• The middle finger bends at the second joint, and the first joint--where the shank rests.
• The first finger is extended forward, both joints slightly bent--the shank rests at the first joint.

B. Move the Scissors to its Resting Place
• Pull your middle finger in toward the palm of the hand, sliding the scissors to the V" of your thumb-- the resting place.
• Your first finger goes along and helps direct the cutters to the "V".

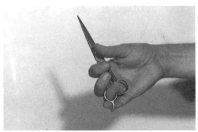

• Keep your ring finger stationary it acts as a pivot point for the scissors' trip.
• The tang slides out till it's positioned between the little finger's tip and first joint.
•Extend your thumb forward and clamp down on the scissors, holding it firmly, but not tightly.
•The first and middle fingers can relax

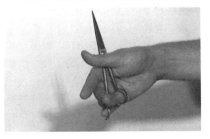

C. Grasping the Comb

•Extend the thumb and first two fingers.
•Grasp the comb.

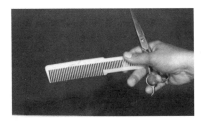
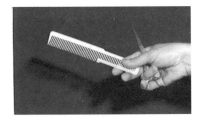

4.4 THE BASIC HAND-TOOL MANIPULATION

Work slowly at first. With practice the nine steps of this basic manipulation will flow together and seem like one quick movement. To explain all the steps that go into one bulk-removal cut, we'll examine the first cut in an equal-length haircut. Wet the hair and comb it forward on top.

***

I hear and I forget. I see and I remember. I do and I understand.   Chinese proverb

Everybody is ignorant, only on different subjects.   Will Rogers

STEP I

Insert comb about one inch into the hair, with the teeth lightly scraping the scalp. Hold the comb flat on the scalp.

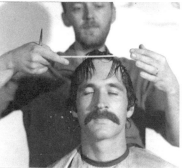

From your view-point it looks like this.

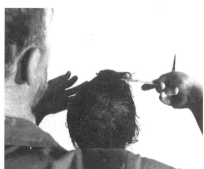

STEP 2

Lift the comb and hair straight up from the scalp. Leave some hair protruding above the comb. Hold the comb in that position.

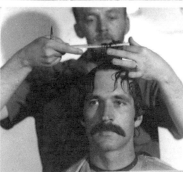

The way you see it.

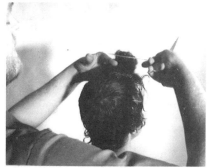

STEP 3 As the last photos show, while you lift up the hair, the left hand is ready to grasp the hair. Position the hair between the holding fingers, below the comb.

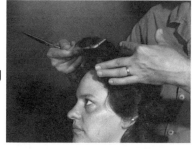

The little and ring fingers (the "spacer fingers") are positioned so the desired length is achieved.

Exactly where the hair is grasped depends on the length you intend to leave the hair. Chapter 6 tells how to make this decision, and section 9 in this chapter has practice exercises that enables you to repeat the same length producing position each time the hair is grasped.

Once the hair is in hand, the holding fingers apply a pinching pressure and a slight upward tug on the hairs to keep them standing straight out from the scalp.

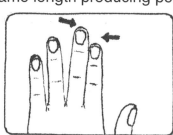

The first and middle fingers, are held in this position.

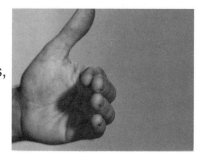

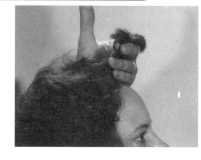

If the holding fingers are on top of each other, the hair isn't held straight out as it should be.

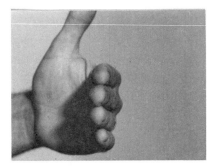
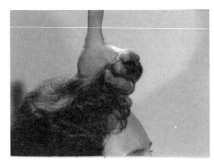

STEP 4 Lift the comb up through the hair above your holding fingers. Then transfer the comb to the "V" of your left hand thumb, and hold the comb there.

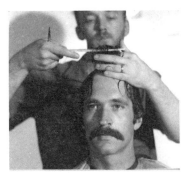
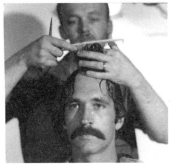
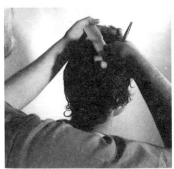

The comb's tip sticks out 2 to 3 inches from the "V" of the thumb.

Combing   The transfer

With practice you'll have enough speed to grasp the hair as the comb makes a nonstop journey up through the hair, to the "V" of the thumb.

STEP 5 Move the scissors from its resting position to the cutting position.

• Pull in your little finger (it's on the tang) as you. .
• Hold your ring finger (in the finger grip) stationary.
• The blades slide out and stop at the first joint of the middle and first fingers.

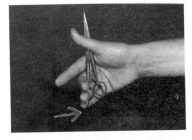
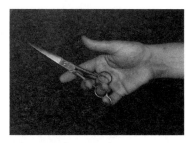

Insert the thumb in its grip and open the blades.

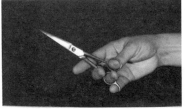
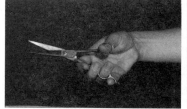
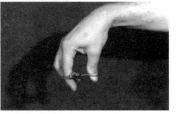

Insert thumb   The cutting position

The ring finger is bent at the second joint and is positioned in the grip at the first joint, which is also bent. The first two fingers are also bent, with the shank positioned at their

***

A man is rich in proportion to the things he can afford to let alone.   Henry David Thoreau

first joint. The thumb is placed in its grip between the tip and the first joint: any farther and it's hard to slip the thumb out again. If it isn't in far enough, you won't have good control as the blades are being opened or closed (an <u>important</u> safety consideration). **STEP 6** Position the blades on both sides of the held hair.

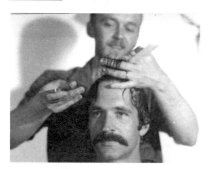 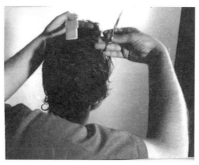 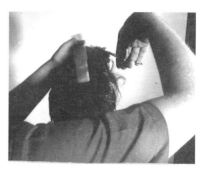

With practice you'll combine this step with step 5. While positioning the scissors in your tool hand, position your arm and wrist so the blades are on both sides of the held hair. Always start cutting at the finger tips and continue toward the big knuckle of the holding fingers. For support, rest the bottom of the thumb blade on the top of the middle finger that is holding the hair. The cutting can be done without this resting guide, but the chances of snipping your holding fingers are increased.

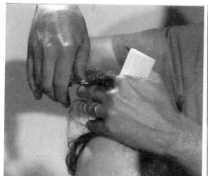 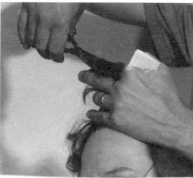

Position the blades flat on top of the holding fingers

Do not position the blades these ways

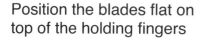

STEP 7 Cut slowly and carefully. it may take a couple of snips to get from the finger tips to the "V" of the holding fingers. You have better control if you make two or even three cuts instead of trying to do it in "one full swoop."

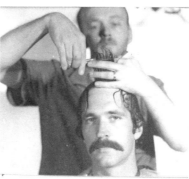

Maintain your holding hand position with the pinching pressure (between the holding fingers) after you have cut the hair.

STEP 8 Return the scissors to its resting place. With the scissors closed, remove the thumb from the thumb grip. The middle finger (which is still bent around the shank at the first joint) pulls the scissors into the resting position at the "V" of the thumb. The ring finger is a stationary pivot point during the trip. The tang should be positioned between the little finger's tip and the first joint when the scissors is at rest. As you reach for the comb, extend the thumb and first two fingers to grab the comb.

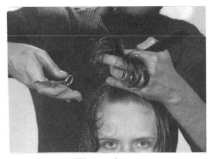 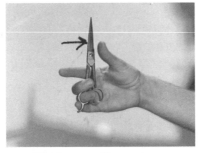 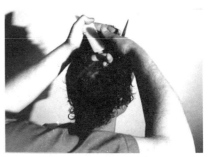

| Thumb out. | To the resting place. | Reach for comb. |

Throughout this step, maintain the position of the left hand with the pinching pressure applied between the two holding fingers.

STEP 9 The tool hand takes the comb from its resting place in the left hand. Pivot the bottom of the left hand away from you while maintaining the pinching pressure. Position the comb at the base of the held hair (teeth lightly scraping the scalp). Slide the comb toward you about an inch, and at the same time, release the hair between your holding fingers. Now comb up another tuft of hair and repeat the basic manipulation.

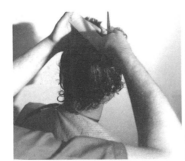 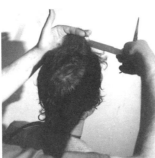 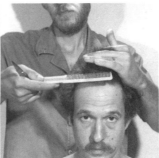 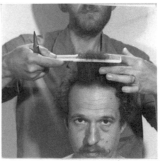

Grab the comb   Pivot bottom of hand and reposition comb   Release and comb up

Holding the hair until you are ready for the next comb up and cut, eliminates snagging the comb in the hair and it insures that you stay on the same pathway, cut after cut. In time you'll gain enough speed to lift your left hand up and release your grip on the hair, while the comb is slipped into position for the next comb up. Until then, the pivot movement gets the job done as you are building speed.

4.5 THE COMB-AWAY METHOD: THE OTHER WAY TO DO IT

This variation of the basic manipulation is necessary to learn because the comb always has to move through the hair, going either against or sideways to the hair grain. If the comb moves through the hair in the same direction as the grain, all you do is comb the hair down--your hand can't grasp the hair if it's combed down.

I find this way of handling the tools is the best (most comfortable and effective) way to do the cutting on the customer's upper left side.

***

Rules for living: Have your yesterdays filed away; your present in order; and your tomorrows subject to instant revision.   Anonymous

Ulcers come from mountain climbing over mole hills.   Anonymous

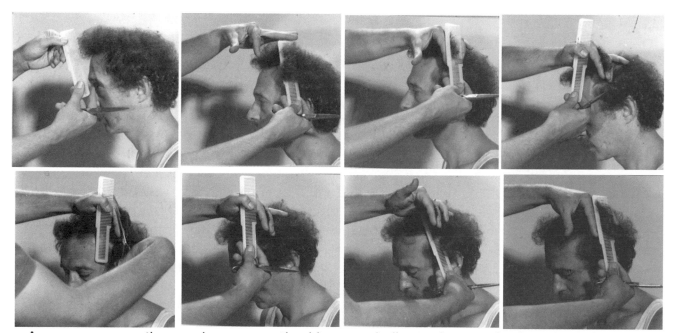

As you can see, the comb-away method is very similar to the standard method. The minor differences are:

• The teeth of the comb point, and the tool hand moves away from you.

• When the comb is in its resting place, the teeth point away from the "V" of the thumb.

• When you insert the comb at the base of the hair held by the left hand, you can see exactly where the comb is placed. Also, you don't need to pivot that hand up to get the comb to the base of the held hair.

This way to use the tools requires <u>extra care</u> because the points of the scissors move toward the head or face, especially when the cutters are in their resting place and you are manipulating the comb. Go slow and be aware of the points of the scissors as they move about. (I've never had any problem, but I am always mindful of where those points are while the comb is being used--you do the same.)

4.6 THREE AIDS TO EQUAL-LENGTH CUTTING

Now that you know how to manipulate hands and tools for one cut in the bulk-removal process, you are ready to learn how to do all the haircut's basic manipulations so the job gets done right. First is the **primary** aid toward the goal of a consistent length to the hair.

<u>Aid 1</u> With every cut made in the bulk-removal process, the bottom of your left hand rests on the scalp.

Something to lean on   Not floating in space

Different cutting lengths require different holding hand positions:

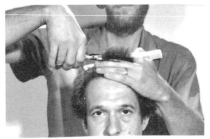 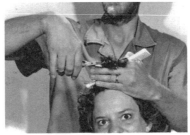 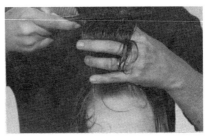

| 1 inch cut | 2 inch cut | 3 inch cut |

The shorter the hair is cut, the closer the fingers of the holding hand are spaced and the more your palm of the hand touches the head. On the shortest version, the inside of the spacer fingers are also touching the scalp. The longer the hair is left, the farther apart the two spacer fingers on your left hand are positioned, and the palm doesn't touch the head--just the bottom edge of the hand and little finger is in contact.

The **important** thing to keep in mind when giving an equal-length haircut is: choose a length for the hair, find the holding hand position that produces that length when you cut, then repeat the same holding hand position throughout the bulk-removal process. (Chapter 7 shows how the hair's length can be altered, but this rule is the **key** to equal-length haircutting.) The practice exercises at the end of this chapter enable you to repeat the same length-producing position, time after time, on the basis of how it feels.

Aid 2 You will be following a systematic sequence of cuts in the pathways and sections of the head. With this system you can't miss a hair on the head. Skim through chapter 7 to see how you go about it.

Aid 3 An advantage of cutting hair in pathways is that you usually work beside a pathway that has already been cut--this cut hair is the hair you use as a guide. You comb up and hold a little of the already-cut hair--the guide-hair--along with the hair to be cut.

For example, say all the cuts are completed in the first pathway.

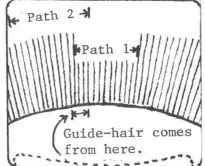

In path two, the comb picks up a little of the shorter, already cut hair from the first path.

The scissors point to the already-cut guide-hair from the first pathway, showing at the "V" of the holding fingers. The longer hair that protrudes above the holding fingers is the uncut hair from the second pathway.

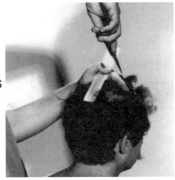

Because of the sequence of paths you cut on the top section, the guide-hair shows at the "V" of the holding fingers on some paths, and at the finger tips on other paths. As you work on the sides and back, guide-hair always appears at the 'V".

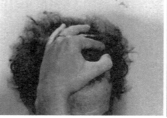 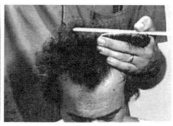

Guide-hair at the "V"   At finger tips

When your left hand is in the correct length-producing position, there should be about 1/8 to 1/4 inch of guide-hair protruding above the holding fingers--cut the longer, uncut hair to match the shorter, already-cut guide-hair. Be sure not to cut any of the guide-hair. There are two main advantages to using the guide-hair aid:
• It keeps you on the right path, making it impossible for you to drift around the head.
• It shows you how much to cut off on the basis of how much was cut off on the last pathway. However, remember the most important way to achieve a consistent length with each cut, is for you to have the bottom of your holding hand in contact with the scalp--this allows you to manipulate that left hand on the basis of *how it feels*.

4.7 MISCELLANEOUS HAND AND TOOL INFORMATION

1. The Holding Hand.

When giving an equal-length hair-cut, pull the hair <u>straight</u> up and out from the head.

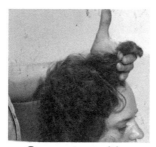 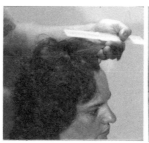

Correct position   Incorrect positions

2. Pulling tension. Be sure all the hairs between your holding fingers are held with a slight pull-up tension that keeps all the hair straight.

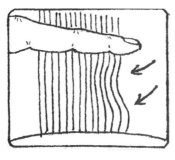

Maintain a gentle upward pressure so no hairs buckle.

Those buckled hairs would have a longer length than those hairs held straight.

Working on curly and kinky hair. With straight or wavy hair the amount of pull out pressure on the held hair can vary from a little to a lot and it won't make any difference. Curly and kinky hair are like coiled springs and must have the same pull out pressure, cut after cut.

It is important that you maintain (as much as possible) the same upward pulling tension on curlier hair, cut after cut. Without a consistent pull out pressure, the hair is cut to uneven lengths.

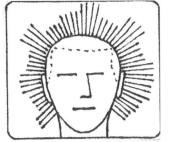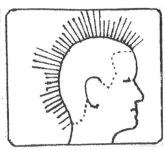

This unevenness can be removed during the second-time-through part of the haircut, but at that time you should just be cutting off minor differences in length.

4. The holding hand conforms to the shape of the head. When the hair is left longer, the bottom of the left hand and little finger rest on the scalp; when the hair is cut to a length of 2 inches or less, more of the palm of the hand and the inside of the little finger (and ring finger too on extra short lengths) rest on the scalp. These shorter lean-on-the-head positions result in the hand conforming to the shape of the head: the holding fingers effortlessly conform too.

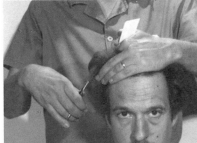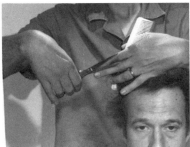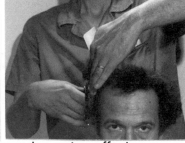

Correct position is relaxed   Incorrect positions require extra effort

The way the left hand conforms to the head depends on the shape of the head in the area you're working on. Heads come in all shapes with some parts of the head fairly flat, and some relatively curved areas. These are the four flatter areas:

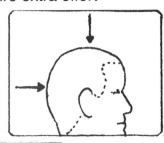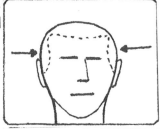

The five curved areas:

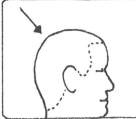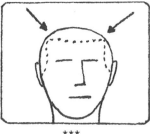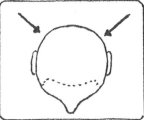

***

There are some men who, in a fifty-fifty proposition, insist on getting the hyphen too.

Dr. Laurence J. Peter

Those who are too smart to engage in politics are punished by being governed by those who are dumber.

Plato

On the flat areas the holding fingers are held more straight; on the curved areas, those fingers conform to the curves by being slightly curved.

On curved parts of the head, fingers are slightly rounded.

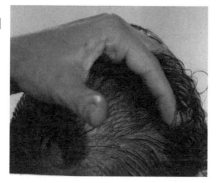

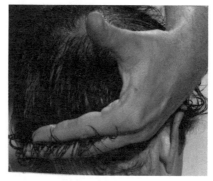

On flat parts of the head, fingers are held straighter.

Relax your hand, and the holding fingers conform effortlessly to the underlying shape of the head. If you have difficulty getting your hand to conform to the curved areas of the head, you could always cut an extra pathway between the two already-cut pathways on the curved area. For example:

When cutting the top of the head--an area of both flat and curved surfaces--you cut the first few paths with ease. On the fourth path there is a curved surface and your holding hand doesn't conform as it should.

After cutting pathway 4, you find the hair is left longer than it should be. To get this hair all the same length, cut an extra pathway between paths 2 and 4. This extra path overlaps both of the two already-cut paths.

Pathways 2 and 4 serve as guide-hair for the hair that needs to be cut. The guide-hair shows at the "V" and tips of the fingers. Cut the longer hairs between the two guide. hairs. (See the photos for the top pathways in chapter 7, section 4-A for more on this.)

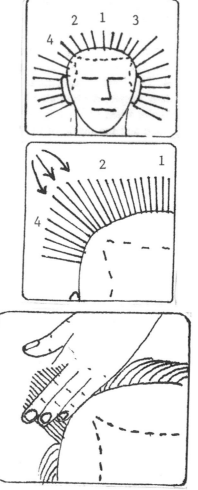

Most beginners are able to get their left hand to conform to the curved areas; if you have problems, just make an extra path between the two already-cut paths, as shown above.

5. The impact of the head shape.

Because the left, holding hand conforms to the shape of the head, the head's shape determines the overall cutting shape--the cutting line you give to the hair. There is a wide variety of head shapes and each shape produces a somewhat different cutting line on an equal-length haircut.

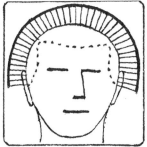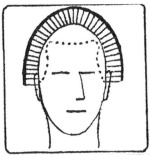

To determine head shape, spend a minute before the haircut, combing through the hair. Pay close attention to the path the comb takes as it travels through the hair. This combing tells you the shape of the head hidden by the hair. A skull may have minor bumps such as the knowledge bump located at the back of the head where the spine meets the skull. Ignore these small irregularities.

6. The Comb and Easy Hair Handling

A. Untangling the hair. Be sure the hair is free of tangles and snarls by thoroughly brushing and combing before cutting. The comb must be able to move through the hair without obstructions. To achieve this you may have to give damaged hair an approximate haircut (see section 8). This procedure removes most of the damaged ends that slow you down, and it makes things less painful for your customer.

B. Combing out the hair. Before starting to cut paths through the hair, always comb through the entire head of hair. This combing is directed away from the crown-area cowlick--the top is combed toward the front, with the sides and back combed downward.

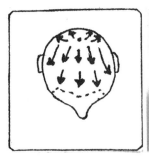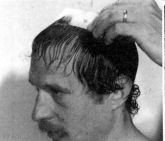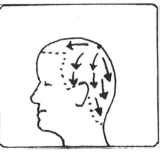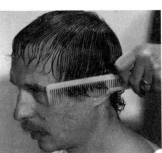

After finishing the cuts in a pathway, always re-comb the hair in the area just cut, before starting the next pathway. Combing the hair this way has the hair lying with the hair grain for the most part. When you make the cuts in the pathways, the sequence of cuts goes in the opposite direction (against the hair grain.) This approach makes it easy to comb the hair out from the head so the left hand can grasp it.

C. What to do when the comb gets snagged. When the comb travels through the hair either going against or sideways to the hair grain, it may get snagged in the hair. Having a pinching pressure between the holding fingers until the comb is reinserted into the held hair eliminates most snag problems during the pathway cutting; but beginning a new pathway can present problems. These aids get you going without snags.

•The helping-hand method. Use this approach when beginning a pathway or whenever your comb snags. When the comb runs onto some uncooperative hair, place your left hand in front of the snag (or below it if the snag is around the sides or back).

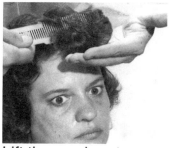

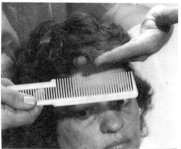

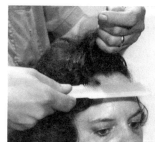

The hand lifts up the hair so the comb can be placed at the base of the held

Lift the comb out and toward the left hand

The hair flops into the palm of the hand

The comb is reinserted

A variation of this method is to grab the edge-lying hair with the left hand, lift it up, and insert the comb at the base of the held hair. If the comb lifts out without snags, you can proceed. If it snags, repeat the helping-hand method shown above, and you're on your way.

• The sideways trick. With this technique you can start out anywhere on a head of hair. It's extra useful when you start the pathways above the ears, (the tops of the ears are easy to catch with the comb if you do it any other way.) Place the comb so that the teeth touch the scalp.

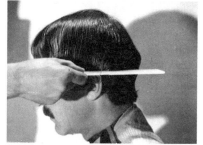

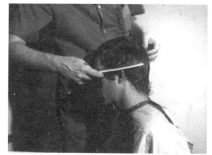

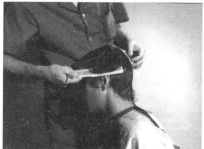

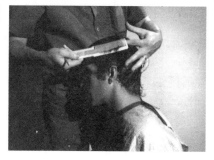

Gently scrape the teeth against the scalp as you move the comb a couple of inches to the left or right

Lie the comb flat (parallel to the head) and insert it about an inch into the hair

Lift the comb away from the head. The left hand grasps the hair before the comb is out of the hair

This procedure works well; however, there may be times when the comb gets snagged as you start the lift-out--use the helping-hand method shown above.

7. Scissors Handling

A. Cutting curly and kinky hair. Straight and slightly wavy hair stand straight out from the holding fingers, making it easy to position the scissors' blades on both sides of the held hair. Curlier hair is less cooperative because it likes to wrap around the tops of your holding fingers. The remedy is simple enough, but somewhat time-consuming. All you do is gently (very gently) scrape the tops of your holding fingers with the points of the blades as the scissors slide into its cutting position. This insures all the held hair gets between the scissor blades.

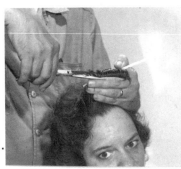 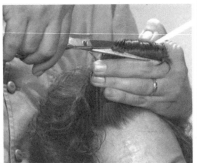 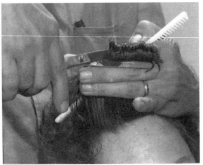

Curly hair requires this slower scissors handling.

B. Positioning. To wield the scissors effectively and comfortably, the wrist should be bent and your arm held away from the body for the top cutting. For best vision on the top cutting, the chair should be in a high position.

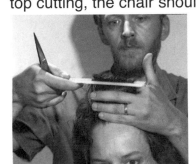

The arm is more relaxed for the cutting on the sides and back. A low chair position is needed for the sides and back.

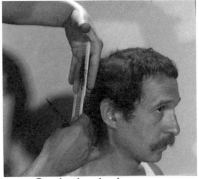

Extra help comes by moving their head to positions more comfortable for you--it may be a little tiring on the neck to hold their head to one side or the other for a period of time, but customers understand your ease in handling the tools is the important consideration, (they do want the best possible haircut.)

4.8 THE OPTIONAL STEP: AN APPROXIMATE HAIRCUT

If you need to cut off a lot (2 to 3 inches or more) of hair, the hair should be made easier to handle before beginning the bulk-cutting. This can be accomplished by using the familiar basic tool manipulation to cut the hair at 10 to 15 evenly spaced locations around the head. I prefer this quicker way of doing it:

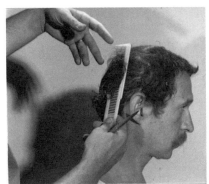 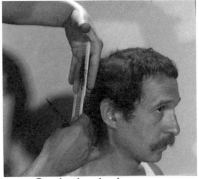 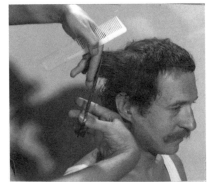

| Insert comb and lift out | Grab the hair below the comb | Comb to resting place; position scissors and cut |

***

My life is in the hands of any fool who makes me lose my temper.   Anonymous

The last photo shows the hair being cut above the holding fingers; it could also be cut on the inside part of the fingers. Be sure to leave the hair at least an inch longer than what is wanted for the final length on the bulk-removal. If the hair needs approximate cutting, you may also want to give it a preliminary edge-cutting (see the next chapter.)

4.9 PRACTICE MAKES PERFECT

Let's say you decide to learn to drive an automobile. How do you go about joining the ranks of the car drivers? You would probably enroll in a driver's education course and get as much practice as you can. This book is your "driver's education" and here is the practice for bulk-cutting skills.

While cutting hair you'll position and move your hands and arms in a variety of ways that are quite unfamiliar. This means you'll start slowly and feel awkward (just like it was when you learned how to drive). The following exercises minimize the awkwardness, and help build muscles, coordination, and speed. If you can, spend an hour a day for a week, getting comfortable with the skills in these exercises--it is time well spent.

The first two exercises train you to hold the left hand in whatever hair length-producing position you may want. With practice, the feel of your hand tells you it's positioned correctly. Use one or both of these first two exercises; each has its own advantages.

Exercise 1 The Practice Board. Get two pieces of plywood or any kind of scrap wood about 1 foot square. Drill a 1/4 inch hole in the center of each. Take two pieces of cord or heavy string about 6 inches long and tie a knot in one end of each. Feed the strings through the holes in the boards.

Using a ruler, mark off 1/2 inch intervals on the strings with two felt-tip pens. Alternate the colors; i.e., every half inch is marked in blue, and every inch is done with a red pen.

Use clay or putty to build up a curved surface on one of the boards. The board with the clay on it simulates the curved areas of a head; the board without the clay represents flatter areas of a head.

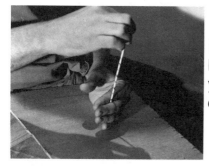

Use your tool hand to hold the string out, while the holding hand grabs the string over and over again-until you are 100 percent familiar with how the hand feels at different length-producing positions.

Practice at all the 1/2 inch marks between 1 and 3 1/2 inches. The advantage of this exercise is you don't take up someone's time as you do with the second and third

58

exercises--you can just sit and fiddle with your strings whenever you like. The next two practice exercises bring more realism into your preparation efforts.

Exercise 2 Comb and Ruler. Here you practice the basic hand-tool manipulation, and a little of the comb-away method as the sequence of cuts are followed for an equal-length haircut's bulk-removal. Instead of handling the scissors you'll have a ruler on a nearby table. As the sequence of cuts are followed, each time the hair is combed up and the hand is in the length-producing position you want, reach for a ruler and measure the results.

Be sure to measure to the top of the first finger in these two places:

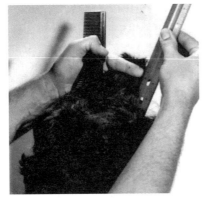 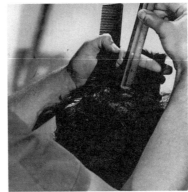

Once or twice through all the cuts should enable you to consistently manipulate the left hand into the desired length-producing position.

Exercise 3 The Dry Run With this exercise you polish your holding hand skills, but also get practice with hands, scissors, and comb working together. Go to Chapter 7 and follow the step-by-step photos of the bulk-removal and second-time-through cutting. Practice every cut as if you were giving a haircut, but close the scissors in front of the hair held by the left hand. Also, practice the helping hand and sideways comb handling methods--use as needed as you go through the bulk cutting.

Take the time to get adept at the tool handling in this chapter. Millions have learned how to use tools this way, you can too.

***

If you don't know where you're going, you will probably end up somewhere else.
Laurence J. Peter

Stay curious.
Motto of my local P.B.S. station

Those who cannot remember the past are condemned to repeat it.   George Santayana

Since the beginning of time each generation has fought nature. Now in the span of a single generation, we must turn and become the protector of nature.   Jacque Cousteau

If you were on trial for being a Christian (Buddhist, Moslem, Hindu, etc.,) would there be enough evidence to convict you?
Anonymous

Thinking is the talking of the soul with itself.   Plato

When I get to be a psychologist, I'll direct all my patients to go and make something with their hands and give it away.
Anonymous

CHAPTER 5 EDGE-CUTTING AND OTHER SKILLS

5.1 EDGE-CUTTING USES A DIFFERENT APPROACH

Edge-cutting (also called edging) is quite different from bulk-cutting. Here you comb the hair down and cut a little hair close to the skin.

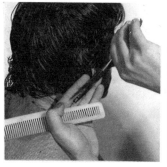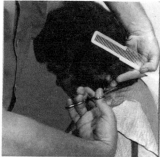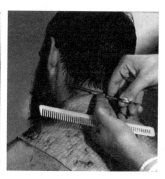

With the bulk-removal done before the edging, the hair around the edges are already shortened from that bulk cutting. Because of this, usually a minimum cutting is all that's needed to get the edge hairs in good shape.

5.2 MAIN RULE FOR EDGE-CUTTING

While there are some differences in the edge-cutting done on the three more advanced haircuts, the main rule for cutting edge hair on an equal-length haircut gives a good introduction to the way the hands and tools are used on all four haircuts. When doing the edging on the equal-length cut, the hair is combed down and out, straight away from the hairline, and your cutting line conforms to the shape of the underlying hairline. In other words, the edge-line cuts are parallel to the underlying hairline. To do this, you must be aware of the shape of the hairline that lies beneath and above the edge hair being worked on.

***

The highest form of wisdom is kindness.

Amish saying

Comb the hair back, up and away from the hairline to see it. Always take the time to see the shape of the hairline.

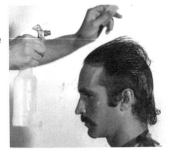
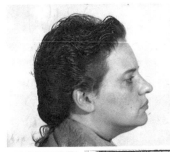

This is a typical hairline:

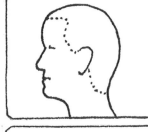
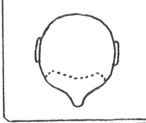
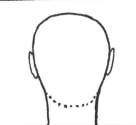

However, there are wide variations from the typical. Here are some of the many less common hairlines:

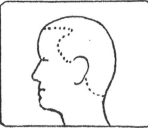
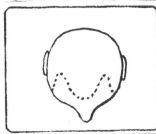
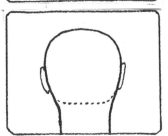

Here the heavy line represents the edge-cutting line; the dashed line represents the underlying hairline:

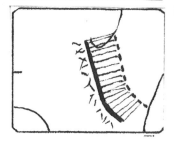
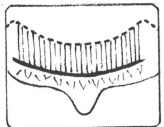
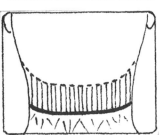

The edge-cutting line conforms to the hairline

There are a few minor exceptions to the main rule for edging:

• Hair covering the ear.
If your cutting conforms to the shape of the hairline in this area, you'll have the edge-line shown on the first illustration. Some like it this way, however, most prefer the edge-line shown on the right.

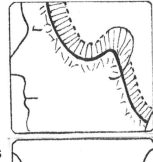
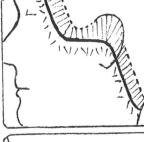

• Neck edge-line.
Besides the common straight across neckline shown above, many have a wavy shape (with a ducktail and a Type 2 hair grain). The edge-line can be cut to conform to the wavy shape but most prefer a straight line.

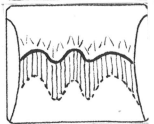
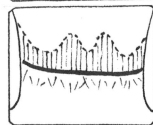

•**Bangs**. Forehead hair is normally cut to conform to the shape of the hairline.

Looking down on the top front of the head, these drawings show the cutting line following the hairline:

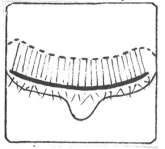 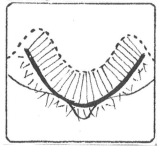 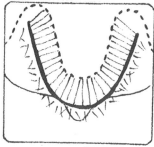

On top hair that grows straight forward (about 15 to 20 percent of the time,) edging can be done as shown above, or a couple of other approaches can be used.

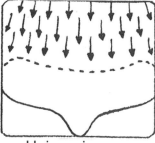 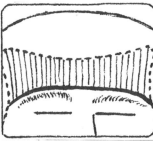 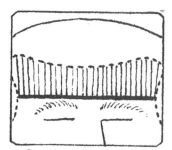

| Hair grain goes forward on top | Edge-line conforms to shape of eyebrows | Or, the edge-line is cut straight across |

5.3 THE TWO TIMES TO CUT HAIR AROUND THE EDGES

Usually the edge hair is cut once, sometimes twice during a haircut.

1. Preliminary cutting. This edging is done only if there is a lot (2 to 3 inches or more) of hair to cut off. This cutting makes the bulk-removal easier--that excess hair is hard to handle, and a minute or two spent cutting around the edges beforehand is time well spent. The same cutting methods are used for this edging as for the final edging. The difference here is the hair is left at least an inch longer than what is wanted for the finished length on the edges--a little margin for error that is taken care of during the bulk-cutting and on the final edge-cutting.

2. Final edging. This edge-cutting is almost always done after the bulk-removal and the second-time-through (smooth it off) cutting is finished. The next section explains why it isn't always necessary, and the last chapter's section on cutting children's hair tells when it's best to avoid cutting the edge hairs. However, the finished product is improved when the edges are trimmed a little.

5.4 HOW MUCH TO CUT OFF?

With preliminary edging you may have to cut off quite a bit of hair; most of the final edging has you cutting off as little hair as possible. This minimum cutting means just snipping off the edge hairs that are a little longer than the majority of edge hairs. If more needs to be cut, usually less than 1/8 inch is sufficient. To explain why a minimum cutting approach is used, you need to know what happens with equal-length bulk-cutting.

Assume the bulk-removal left the hair 2 inches long all over. Comb the hair into the edge-cutting position and the tips of those hairs that grow at the hairline now lie 2 inches from the hairline.

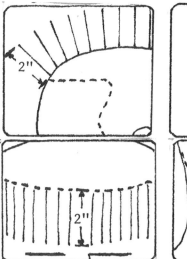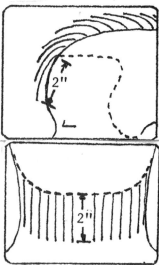

The same holds true anywhere on the head of hair--the hair ends lie 2 inches from the hairline anywhere the hair is combed straight away from the hairline.

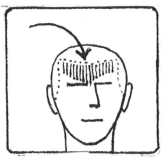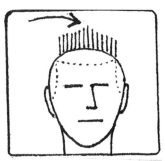

With a smooth bulk-cutting, the tips of the edge hairs are parallel to the hairline they are combed away from--they're already in the basic shape you want when the main rule for edge-cutting is followed. (This is why the edging can be skipped, if you give a haircut to a child who can't sit still.)

If the hair wasn't cut evenly on the bulk-removal, when the hair is combed down for edging there will be some extra long hairs. Go back through that area and redo the bulk-cutting--the long hairs are gone when the hair is combed down a second time.

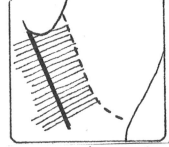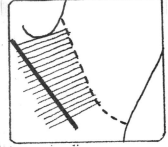

Because the bulk-removal is smoothed off by the second-time-through cutting, there is little chance to find edge hairs as uneven as shown above. Nevertheless, if some edge hairs are found to be longer than their neighbors, check to be sure the bulk-cutting in that area was done right. Assuming the edge-line is free of bulk-removal boo-boos, only cut off the small number of hairs that are a bit longer than the majority of hairs on the edges--a little smoothing off does it.

The heavy, solid lines represent edge-cutting lines on the side of the neck:

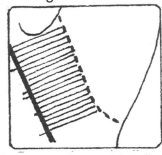

Correct edge-cutting line   Incorrect edge-cutting lines

***

Inflation is when you pay $5.00 for the $2.00 haircut you use to get for $1.00 when you had hair.

Franklin P. Jones

Going back to the example of the two-inch equal-length haircut, if an inch of length is cut off the edge hair, you would undo your bulk-cutting efforts. Cutting edge hair one-inch shorter creates the unevenness shown in the far illustration.

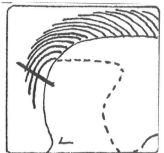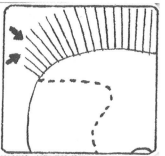

If the edge hair needs to be cut a little shorter than just trimming off the long ones, stay within these guidelines:

Bulk-removal length	How much can be cut
1 inch	1/8 inch
2 inches	1/4 inch
3 inches	3/8 to 1/2 inch

There are three exceptions to the above guidelines--these areas offer some flexibility:

1. Neckline hair. If you've given a 3 inch haircut to a person with a short neck, and the three inches of hair below the neck's hairline does not fit the person well, or if they prefer not to have the neck hair brushing against their collar, as much as 2 inches of the neck hair can be cut off. If the neckline hair is cut an inch (or more) shorter, some tapering is needed to avoid a bowl-cut appearance to the neck hair (see chapter 6 for the 2-step tapering procedure).

2. Hair in front of and covering the ear. Here you may need to cut off 1/2 inch (or more) of the perimeter hair in order to have the straight across edge line that was shown earlier in this chapter. If an inch of this ear-area edge hair is cut off, it will also need a little 2-step tapering to have the hair lie well.

3. Lower temple-area hair. If you give a longer version of the equal-length cut, the lower temple region hair may have to be cut shorter than the minimum approach. This hair can flop forward into the corners of the eyes if left too long.

5.5 BULK-CUTTING AND ITS IMPACT ON BANGS AND EAR-AREA HAIR

For the guidelines below to hold true, assume the hair being cut is straight and fine-textured with a Type 1 hair grain. Understand that these lengths are approximates: factors such as a receding or low hairline, big or small ears, all have an influence on these averages. After you have done the bulk-cutting that leaves these lengths, you can expect the hair to lie as shown.

Bulk-removal length	Hair covering the ears	Bangs
3 inches	To bottom of the ears or slightly longer	To about the eyebrows or a little longer
2 inches	About 1/2 or more of the ear covered	About 1/2 to 2/3 of the forehead covered
1 inch	Top 1/4 or less of ear covered	Hair lies 1/5 to 1/4 down the forehead

As the next section indicates, these approximate lengths don't hold true when working on some kinds of hair other than straight, fine, Type 1 hair.

5.6 THE EDGE-LINE WILL SHRINK

The edge-line likes to raise up, and appear to have shrunk, when you're giving the hair a final look-over at the end of the haircut. Several different factors can cause this--when two or more are present, expect major shrinkage.

A. The Springy Nature of Wavy, Curly, Kinky Hair

The curlier types of hair are usually pulled down into a cutting position. After the cutting, they resume their normal (out from the scalp) way of being, and the edge-line raises quite a bit. The curlier the hair, the more it rises up from the cutting position. For example, say a curly head of hair is given a 3 inch cut. When edge cutting on the bangs, the hair is pulled down to eyebrow level. After cutting, the hair is released and it rises up halfway on the forehead. The same result is true for other parts of the edging.

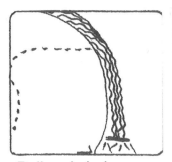 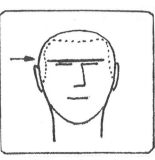 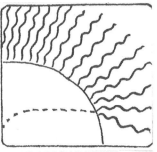 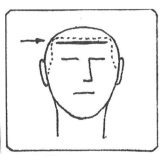

| Pull curly hair to cutting line | After cutting it springs back | Cut curly hair at this point | The edge hairs rise to here or higher |

B. The Direction the Hair Wants to Lie

With curly and kinky hair, hair grain does not have much impact on the lying direction of the hair. Hair grain on straight or slightly wavy hair has a major impact on which way it lies. How this causes the edge-line to shrink is illustrated by the two examples below.

• If the hair has a Type 2 hair grain, it greatly affects where the hair ends up lying as it covers the ear.

For example, say you give a 3 inch equal-length cut. On the edging, the hair is pulled down over the ear--the edge hairs are cut below the ear.

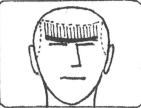

When the hair lies the way it wants, toward the back of the head, the edge line rises almost halfway up the ear.

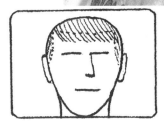

• If the hair grain on the top of the head goes off to one side and the edge-line is cut at eyebrow level, expect the hair to lie almost halfway on the forehead.

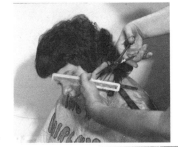

C. Dry Hair Has Body, Wet Hair Does Not
All of your scissors haircutting is done with the hair wet.

Wet hair is softened and weighted down; it lies flat on the skin when it's being cut.

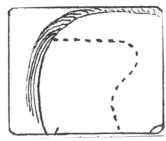

When wet hair dries, the added weight is gone-- the hair has body and the edge line rises.

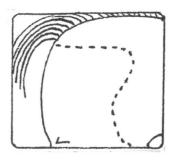

How much this factor causes the hair to shrink up depends largely on the texture of the hair. Fine hair tends to be limp whether it is wet or dry, so there won't be much effect on this hair type. Coarse hair is a different story: if your edging was done to 3 inch long coarse hair, you could expect the hair to shrink up as much as 1 inch. As you can see, where the hair finally lies around the edges is determined by several different factors. With this information an educated guess will usually be right on the mark, but cutting edge hair so it lies exactly where it's wanted requires you to "feel" your way:
•Do not cut off too much edge hair at one time. You can always cut off more hair, so be cautious with the first cutting on the edges..
•Expect to modify the bulk-removal length on the second haircut a person gets. The length the hair is left on bulk cutting determines the length of those edge hairs. First haircuts are a learning experience: make good guesses, but don't be disappointed if it takes a second cutting before you zero-in on the best possible cutting length.

5.7 FOUR EDGING METHODS: HOW TO DO THEM

The bulk-removal involved only two basic hand-tool methods. Edge cutting, while it takes only 10 to 15 percent of your haircutting time, requires four different methods. Don't despair. There are good reasons for this, and because you've already learned the how-to for bulk-cutting, these techniques are quite easy to learn

A. The Modified-Bulk-Removal Method
As the name implies, this edge-cutting is done with the same basic hand-tool manipulation used for bulk-cutting. There are a couple of minor differences:
(1) On bulk-cutting, the hair is combed straight up and out from the scalp. With this edging method, comb the hair more forward (about 45 degrees) and grasp the hair between the holding fingers.

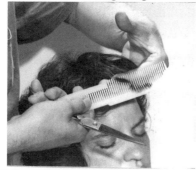

Then pull the hair down and straight away from the hairline. Cut off the hairs longer than the majority.

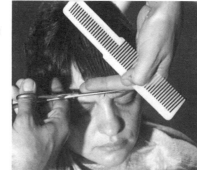

(2) When bulk-cutting, paths are cut through the hair. With this cutting, the top hair is

66

combed from a little behind the hairline, forward away from the hairline, (the sides and back hair is combed down, away from the hairline.) The hair is held by the holding hand, then a small amount of the hair is cut off. Move around the head, repeating this procedure on the neighboring edge hair--the cut hair is a guide for the hair to be cut.

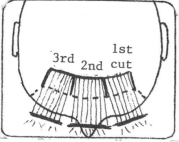 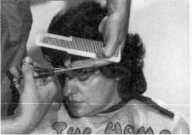 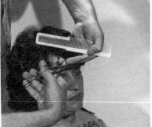 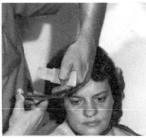

Edge-cutting affects a small part of the hair

Begin at the front, left of the bangs and move around the head

(3) To hold the hair down and away from the hairline, your hair holding hand is used in a slightly different manner than what you're used to. There are three ways to handle the hair; which one is used depends on the length the hair was left during the bulk-removal:

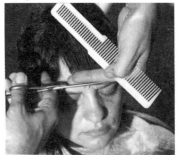

• Medium lengths. If the hair is 2 to 2 1/2 inches long, tuck the spacer fingers in, under the hair being held. The little finger rests against the hairline and helps insure the holding fingers also conform to the shape of the hairline.

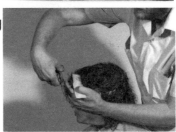

• Longer hair. With hair longer than 2 1/2 inches, slide the holding fingers out on the hair shafts until the desired cutting position is reached. There won't be anything to lean on, so be extra aware of the shape of the underlying hairline, and have the holding fingers conform (be parallel) to it.

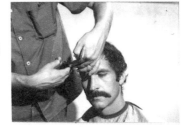

• Shorter hair. When dealing with hair shorter than 2 inches, the spacer fingers can't tuck under the held hair--there isn't enough room. Position the holding fingers so they reflect (are parallel to) the shape of the hairline. Let the inside of the spacer fingers rest on the skin.

This less than 2 inch, more than 2 inch rule is flexible in that it depends on the size of the fingers. Small fingers could go as short as 1 1/2 to 1 3/4 inches with the tuck under approach; big fingers might need more than 2 1/2 inches of length in order to fit those spacer fingers under the held hair. While this kind of edging can be used on most parts of your edge-cutting, I like it mainly for edging around the face, especially the bangs. It leaves the edge hair with a softer appearance than do the next three methods.

B. The Finger-Bracing-the-Scissors Method

This method works well when the hair is on the short side. It can be used on any of the edging except for the hair that covers the ear--the last method is best for that edging. This method is often used to trim the neckline and bangs on the equal-length cut, and it will always be used for trimming men's sideburns. There are two ways to do it:

1. The standard way. The tool hand has the same beginning position for the comb and scissors as used for bulk-cutting. If the bottom neck hair is to be trimmed, comb the hair down, away from the hairline, so the hair lies on the skin. Put the comb in its resting place, and position the scissors in your tool hand for cutting. With the blades open, use the first finger or two of your left hand to support and steady the scissors as the skin is gently scraped with the dull outside part of the thumb blade's point. When the blades are positioned on both sides of the hair to be cut, the point of the thumb blade has slipped under the hair, while the finger blade remains visible.

When the point touches the skin, slide the scissors forward a half-inch or so, and make the cut.

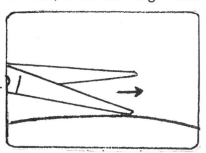
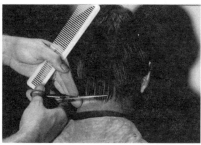

If the hair remains lying in a cutting position, slide the scissors forward for more cutting.

If the hair needs to be combed down again, place the scissors back in its resting position and grab the comb--you're ready for the next comb down and cut.

2. The upside-down way. This approach is the same as the standard way, except that here you can see the back of your hand, while the standard approach has the inside of the hand visible.

This method has the cuts go in the opposite direction than the standard way. Note the different position for the finger that does the bracing.

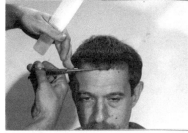
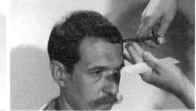

Upside-down   Standard

• As the above photos show, always hold the blades perpendicular to the skin--you want the back of the blade to be in contact with the skin

Never cut with only the point of the blade touching the skin.

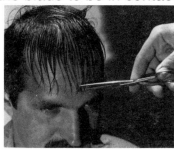

Never cut with the side of the blade in contact with the skin.

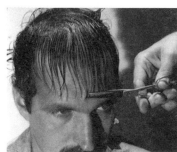

• Cut at a right angle to the hair's combed out, lying position.

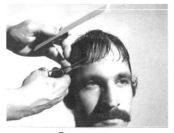 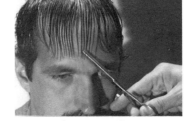

Correct   Incorrect

• Do your cutting with short, half-inch snips rather than one long snip. Make a cut, open the blades, move the cutters forward another half-inch, make another cut, etc. Re-comb whenever the hair gets bent away from its straight out from the hairline lying position.

•As much as possible, the cuts should go against the grain. For example, if the grain goes this way:

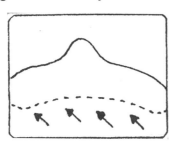

Have the cuts go in this direction:

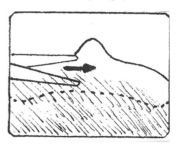

C. The Scissor-and-Comb Method

This way of cutting is useful with shorter hair, especially where the hair's grain is strong enough to prevent the hair from lying straight away from the hairline for the edging you want to do. The comb, handled by the left hand, bends the hair away from its natural lying inclinations as the tool hand manipulates the scissors. There are a couple of steps involved:

• Comb through the hair toward the edge-line for an inch or two. Stop the comb when the ends of the comb's teeth are where you want the edge-line to be--some hairs will protrude from the ends of the comb's teeth.

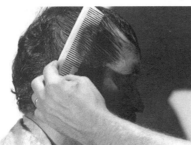 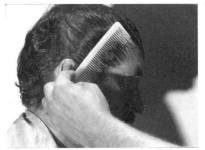 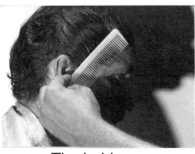

The comb-through   The hold

• With the comb in this holding position, lift the teeth of the comb about 1/4 inch away from the skin while the backbar of the comb is pressed against the hair and scalp. This pivoting movement with the comb pulls the hair that protrude beyond the comb's teeth away from the skin. Now there's ample room to position the scissors blades on both sides of the hair to be cut.

***

Always do right. This will gratify some people and astound the rest.   Mark Twain

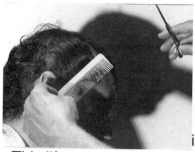 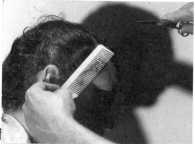 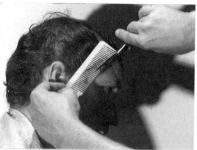

if

This lift-out procedure usually gets all of the hair to be cut, away from the skin for your cutting ease. However, some hairs may slip from the comb--cut the remaining hairs held by the comb, then repeat the comb through and lift-out to get all of those ends cut.

Repeating this a second time needs the use of guide-hair. Look close to see the already-cut hair. The shorter guide-hairs are seen against a background of longer uncut hair.

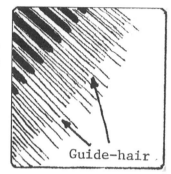
Guide-hair

Stop the comb when the teeth are at the guide-hair. Pivot the comb out, then cut.

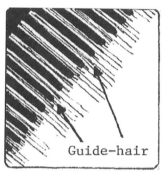
Guide-hair

D. Pull-And-Cut Method

With this edging method, the left hand resumes its role of holding the hair (with a new twist to it,) and the tool hand manipulates both the scissors and comb again. This method works well if the bulk-cutting left the hair 1 1/2 inches long or more. The pull-and-cut can be used on any part of the edge-cutting, but there are three occasions when I find it to be the best way to go: preliminary edging; the edging on the hair that comes down over the ear; and edging longer hair that doesn't want to lie straight away from the hairline. This is how its done:

• Hold the comb and scissors in the tool hand. The teeth of the comb lightly scrape the scalp as you comb through the hair at a right angle to the hairline.

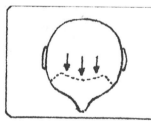 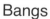 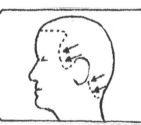 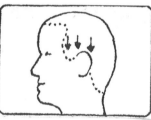 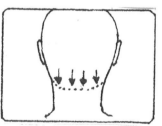

| Bangs | Temple and side of neck hair | Hair in front and covering the ear | Bottom neck hair |

***

Love doesn't make the world go round. Love is what makes the ride worthwhile.

Franklin P. Jones
Robert Browning

Take away love and our earth is a tomb.

The purpose of life is to learn how to love.

Anonymous

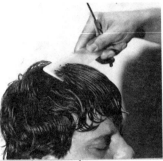
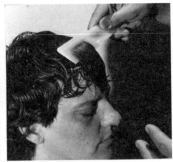
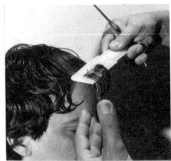

The combing begins several inches back from the hairline.

• As the last photo above shows, as the comb starts scraping the skin (forehead, sides of neck etc.,) tilt the comb away from the skin, as the comb continues through the hair. This combing gives ample room to slip the holding fingers onto the hair.

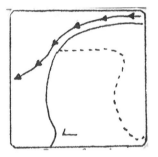
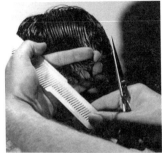

Route of the comb   Hair grasped

•Place the comb in its resting place and apply the pinching pressure between the holding fingers as the fingers slide out to the length-producing position you want. Position the scissors for cutting on the *inside* of the holding hand (this is new twist mentioned earlier.)

These photos show the pull-and-cut used on the side of the neck. Each cut was preceded by the combing described above.

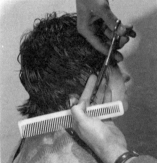
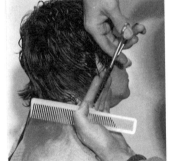
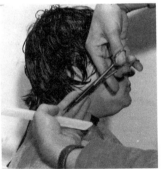

• The middle finger and spacer fingers touch the skin. Cut as close to the hair's lying position as possible.

• Make the cuts on the inside of the hand whenever the pull-and-cut is used. Doing the cutting this way is the **safest** way of using this method. You may notice in the haircut chapters I occasionally do the cutting above my holding fingers. My old habits--this is the way I learned this method a half-a-century ago--show up occasionally when giving longer haircuts. (For the sake of consistency, I would have re-shot those few photos to show the cutting done the right way, but it wasn't possible to get those folks used as models back for a re-shoot.)

***

The art of being wise is knowing what to overlook.   William James

Life is what happens while you are making other plans.   John Lennon

Anyone who stops learning is old, whether at twenty or eighty. Anyone who keeps learning stays young.   Henry Ford

5.8 SEQUENCE OF CUTTING

Like bulk-cutting, edge-cutting needs a systematic approach to have every edge hair cut to the right length. Glance through the edging part of the equal-length haircut chapter; the cutting moves from a cut area to a neighboring uncut area (with minor exceptions) in a specific sequence of cuts all around the the head. Here again, this approach allows the guide-hair aid to be used. Remember to be aware of the shape of the hairline, and have your holding fingers and cutting conform to it whenever possible.

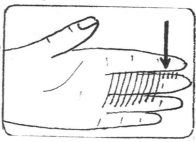
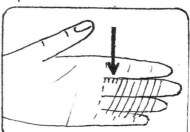

•The preferred pull-and-cut method has the guide-hair show at the fingertips or at the "V" of the holding fingers, depending on what part of the edging you're working on.

When I do the cutting above my holding fingers, my fingers slide out far enough on the hair shafts so the shorter hairs (from the last cut) fall

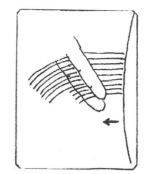
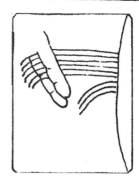

emoval method, one cut alongside of another, the
inary bulk-cutting.
hen using the scissors-and-comb method, overlap the
air from the last scissors-and-comb cutting is included.
guide-hair is at the tips of the teeth. Pivot the comb
g is a continuation of the previous cut.
guide-hair each time you make a short snip and move
s a continuation of the line made by the previous cut.

G

edge-cutting methods you should have already gone
bulk-removal tool handling. This additional practice
0 minutes a day for a few days to go through the
ulk-cutting. Practice all four edging methods, and
eeded to get excellent results on your first equal-

***

to learn.   Greek proverb

thers see stepping stones.   Anonymous

5.10 DRYING THE HAIR

Before getting into the last steps of the haircut, the hair has to be dried. You'll be checking the hair for any less than smoothly-cut areas--heavy, wet hair hides the imperfections. There are a couple of ways to get the hair dried.

A. The Slow Dry
If the hair is to be air-dried, first give the hair a thorough towel-drying. Then comb or brush the hair so it lies with or is only slightly bent away from the hair grain. This comb out is necessary because as the hair air-dries, the hair will "set"--if it's lying in different directions before the air-dry, it does the same after it dries. Slow drying causes a head of wavy hair to become more wavy, even curly, because wet hair clings together--this multiplies the hair's tendency to be wavy or curly. If the person prefers less wavy or curly hair, use a hair dryer, or this next drying method.

B. The Fast Dry
If the customer is in a hurry or they want straighter lying hair, thoroughly towel-dry the hair, then: "Drum dry" the hair with the fingers:

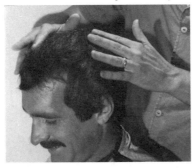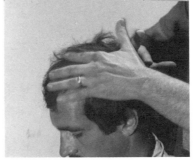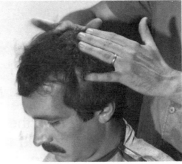

A rapid drumming dries a head of hair in less than a few minutes--when it would have taken as long as a half-hour to air-dry. Of course, even faster drying happens with a hand dryer--include the drum drying with the other hand as the dryer is used. Hand comb the hair into its preferred lying position after it's dry, or nearly so. These faster ways of drying the hair adds extra body and fullness to the hair. If the hair is just air-dried, it is weighted down from the moisture and it sets close to the scalp. When the hair is drummed-dry with or without a hand dryer, it fluffs and dries farther from the scalp. If the hair is flippy after the hair lays the way it wants, this is the time to take care of it.

5.11 HOW TO DEAL WITH FLIPPY HAIR

When I see someone walk in the shop with flippy, misshapen hair, most of the time it is caused by too much length, or uneven cutting. Other causes include wearing the hair so it bends from its preferred way of laying, and things like oiliness and damaged hair. The precision haircuts learned here rule out uneven cutting as a cause for flips, but it only takes a few seconds to check a flippy area to be sure the bulk-cutting has left the hair evenly cut. Use both the first-time-through bulk removal and the second-time-through hand positioning--if uneven cutting is found, trim as needed. If the flippy area is cut right, you can try a little hair bending. A brush with wide-spaced teeth and a spray bottle with warm water will be needed. Wet the hair and brush through the flip area.

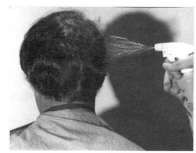
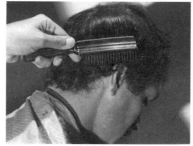
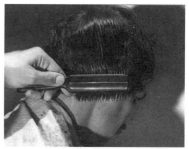
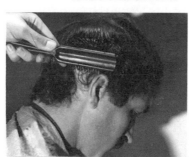
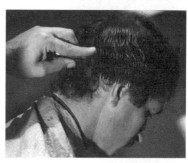
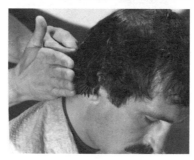
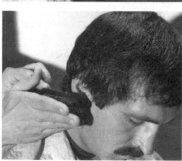

With the teeth of the brush scraping the scalp, brush up through the hair against the hair grain until it is positioned over the flip area. Roll the brush upward and turn it until the teeth point away from the scalp.

Place the other hand over the teeth and continue rolling as the brush is pulled down and out of the hair. This coaxes the hair ends to curve in and lie toward the scalp. Let the hair air-dry in this position and the flips should be gone.

If a hand dryer is used, apply the heat as the brush is being pulled out of the hair.

On some conditions, no amount of "de-flipping" takes care of those stubborn flips:

1. Protruding Ears. The hair that comes over the ears will flip out from the head when ears protrude far enough from the head, and you have not left the hair long enough. This condition affects your decision about the right length to leave the hair during the bulk-cutting. The next chapter describes the remedy.

2. The Nature of the Hair. A lot of folks (mainly men) want their curly hair to be straight. Spend an hour or two trying to de-flip curly hair will be time wasted. Cutting curly hair on the short side is effective: a length of 3/4 to I inch usually has the curls lying into waves. As the hair grows longer, flippy curls are bound to return. Acceptance is a healthy solution to curly hair--hair straightener is the poor alternative.

3. **Hair Grain Problem Areas**. A severe hair grain clash can create the kind of flippy hair that defies any remedy. A small percentage of people have ducktail neck hair that flips out no matter what length it's been left, or how much de-flipping is tried. While fairly rare, you can expect to run across it. Again, acceptance is the only remedy.

Another, more rare kind of clash can "pop up" on the top front hairline: a cowlick in this area may need extra hair length so the hair can bend a little and lie down. More specific information on these subjects is found in the next chapter.

4. Hair Left Too Long. A common flippy condition occurs when Type 2 hair grain combines with fine-textured hair. If this hair is left too long, gravity and the hair's excess weight force the side hair to bend downward, instead of toward the back as the hair grain would like it to lie. Whenever hair doesn't lie the way it wants to, flippy hair is the result. The remedy is simple: cut it shorter.

5.12 PARTING THE HAIR

These rules only apply to straight and wavy hair. Curlier hair types, with their out and away from the scalp way of being, don't lend themselves to a definite part as do the straighter varieties.

A. The Natural Part

Finding the natural part when you have given an equal-length cutting to the top hair is a simple procedure. Comb all of the top hair toward the front. Then start at the front hairline and comb straight back to the crown region.

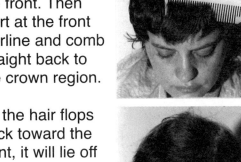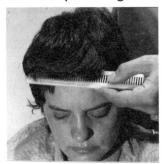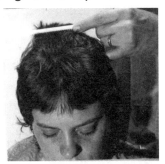

As the hair flops back toward the front, it will lie off to one side or the other, or it may split in the middle, revealing a center part.

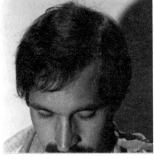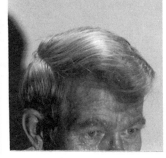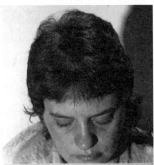

This procedure is best done to hair that has been given a fast drying so that no drying set has influenced the way the hair wants to lie. The equal-length cutting on top is mandatory for finding the natural part because this kind of cutting lets the hair lie as it wants--uneven cutting or the hair left longer on one side of the top hair than the other will have an influence on the way the hair lies. On some heads of hair the top flops straight back toward the front. Hair like this, usually with a Type 1 hair grain and the cowlick located at the center of the crown region, does not have a natural part, but it normally lends itself to the next way to part hair.

B. Forced Parting

To part a head of hair that does not have a natural part, you need to perform the following tool-handling procedure.

First, comb the hair forward, from the cowlick to the front hairline. If it's a center cowlick, there are any number of different paths the comb can take through the hair:

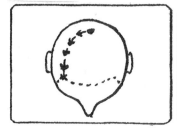 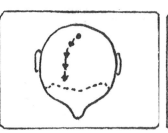 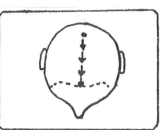 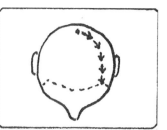

Place the comb in a "comb line" created from the first step. This line must begin in the center of the cowlick, otherwise the cowlick stands on end like a rooster's tail.

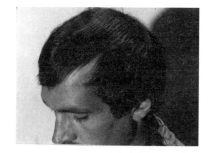 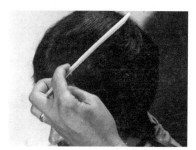

Comb the top hair over the top toward the opposite side as you place your other hand over the side hair. Then hold the top hair with your free hand while you comb the hair below the part down the side. More how-to:

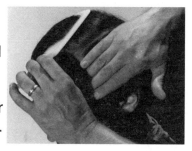 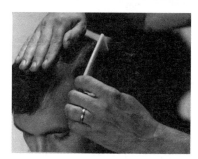

(1) If the cowlick is on the side of the crown region, the hair should be parted on the same side that the cowlick is on. This makes for easier parting and it results in the hair lying according to the grain in almost all cases. The exception is the reverse hair grain described back in the first chapter--this unusual growth pattern needs to have the hair parted on the side of the head that is opposite of the cowlick. Here, the part begins at the cowlick; have it go around the back of the head, and then forward on the other side.
(2) If the cowlick is in the center of the crown region, check to see if the front hair wants to lie toward the left or right--use the hair grain checkout explained in the first chapter. Or you can figure it out by looking for the "big puff"--look closely at how much the hair stands out when it is combed first to one side and then to the other.

For example, if the hair is combed in this direction:

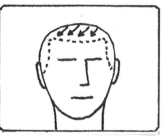

and the hair lies this way:

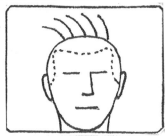

***

Under certain circumstances, profanity provides a relief denied even to prayer. Mark Twain

It is better to know some of the questions than all of the answers. James Thurber

Then the hair is combed in the opposite direction and it lays this way:

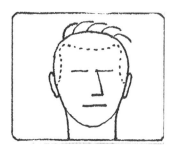

The lay of the hair says the last combing is the way the hair grain wants it to lay. When hair lays with the hair grain, it lays closer to the scalp--comb it against the grain, and it puffs out, farther from the head. In this case, the hair would be parted on the right side of the person's head.

If no "puff" occurs when the hair is combed in both directions, the hair can be parted on either side.

(3) The hair needs to be and parted some-where between the two "V"s on the front hair-line:

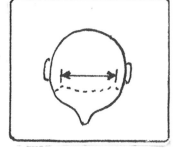

If the hair is parted lower down into the side hair, you're fighting the hair grain and gravity. That side hair wants to lie in a downward direction--it. has to be bent to go up and over the top of the head, plus it always wants to go back to its downward-lying desires.

(4) If there's a cowlick on the front hairline, the part should be made into the center of it. Usually, the hair "falls" into this kind of part by itself. Any other placement of the part would fight the hair grain and have little chance for the hair to lie well.

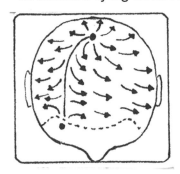

5.13 FINAL LOOK-OVER AND MAKING ADJUSTMENTS

With the hair dried and brushed out you'll be able to see how well the "shingles are lying on the roof'. This is when the hair needs a good looking over to see if any last-minute corrections are needed. Use the back-bar mirror to make the inspection. Ask the following questions:

(1) Are the two sideburns the same length in relation to the ears on both sides? You have to raise up the longer side to match the shorter.

(2) Is the hair covering the ears cut to the same position on both ears? If one ear is more exposed than the other, trim the longer side to match the shorter.

(3) Are there any sloping edge lines? Check it all the way around, but give extra attention to the bangs and neckline. Trim as needed.

(4) Are there any heavy spots in the bulk-cutting? If there is an area that appears heavier than the rest, that heavy spot is caused by hair that is too long. It needs a little recutting to make it the same length as the neighboring hair.

***

It is the chiefest point of happiness that a man is willing to be what he is. Desiderius Erasmus

Justifying a fault doubles it. Anonymous

The longer hair that produces a heavy spot shows up in a couple of ways--as a bulky spot or a line. In either case, go back through that area and use the same hair holding position that was used during the bulk cutting.

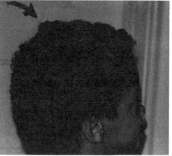
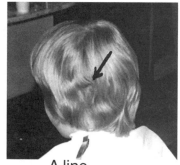

Bulky spot   A line

Where the hair is combed out to get the longer hairs standing out from the head will depend on the kind of hair you're cutting.

• If it's curly or kinky hair, this hair's stand-out-from-the-head nature means the unevenness you see is the place where the comb out happens.

If the heavy spot is here:

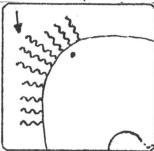

The comb-out and hold for cutting is done right there.

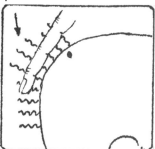

• With wavy or straight hair, the comb must be inserted into the hair at some distance from the line or heavy spot. The reasons for this are: (1) Straighter hair doesn't spring out from the head the way curlier hair does. It lies down, so the ends that cause the heavy spots are at some distance from their roots. (2) To get the hair to stand straight out from the scalp, the comb-out always starts at the roots of the hair that need to be cut.

For example, say you give a 2 1/2 inch hair-cut to a person with straight hair, and a bulky (uneven) spot is found on the side:

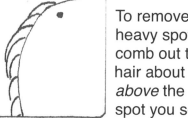

To remove this heavy spot, comb out the hair about 2 inche *above* the heavy spot you see.

If the line or heavy spot is on the top of the head, the comb-out must be done some distance *back* toward the crown region. Whatever hair type you're working on, always comb up and hold some of the neighboring, correctly-cut hair to use as guide-hair. Don't cut any of those guide hairs, just use them.

5.14 CUTTING THE EXTRA, UNWANTED HAIRS

While women don't usually have problems with this, post-adolescent males have hair loss where they would like to keep it, and they grow it in a number of places where they could do without. Maybe it's Mother Nature's way of keeping things in balance?

A. Eyebrow Trimming

Here you need to learn a new way of using hands and tools, called the scissors-over-comb method. It's also used for beard trimming (see that section in the last chapter for more how-to,) or anywhere you want the hair extra short. Now the comb replaces your left hand as a spacer tool. Like your hand, the comb has the function of holding the hair straight out from the skin for the cutting. To achieve this last function, the comb must move through the hair against or at least sideways to the hair grain. When the comb moves that way, the hair builds up and stands out from the skin at the comb's backbar-- where the cutting is done. To trim the brows, you have to know about their grain.

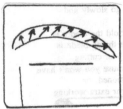 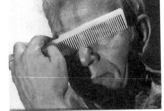 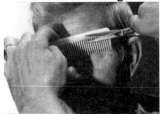

Typical eyebrow grain   Left hand positions comb   Cut protruding hairs

To leave the brows longer, position the comb as shown, then move the comb away from the skin to the desired distance to make the cuts.

B. The Ears

Hair usually crops out on the top edge of the ear and on the little "nubby" located at the front, center part of the ear. This hair can be cut by using a close-cutting clipper (the safest approach,) an electric razor, a safety razor and soap, or a scissors with the finger-bracing method. When this last method was used for edge-cutting, the cutters were held perpendicular to the skin; here the scissors are held at a 45 degree angle (or less) to cut those hairs as short as possible. Always go slow and be sure there isn't any skin between the blades.

C. Nose Hair

If there is such a thing as "unsightly" hair, it has to be a group of hairs protruding from the nose! I always use my close-cutting Finisher clipper for this. The finger-bracing method can be used to cut **only** those hairs that protrude from the nose. Cut the "ugly" hairs very carefully, and never do any cutting inside the nostril--lots of potential for big trouble there. If there are any hairs growing on top of the nose, trim those too.

D. Stray Hairs on the Sides of the Neck and Below the Neckline

Here too, I use a clipper to get rid of these stray hairs. A razor can be used, (preferably a safety razor with shaving lather,) to remove the extra hairs that grow beyond the edge-cutting line. Another approach is to use the scissors-over-comb method that was used to trim eyebrows. This approach, like cutting the brows, leaves the hair cut to a length that is equal to, or a little longer than the thickness of the comb, if the comb is held so it touches the skin. For a longer length, hold the comb at some distance from the skin.

5.15 SAFETY CONSIDERATIONS

Safety is free--it only costs a little time and concern. Be extra generous with it.

A. Relatively Safe Situations

When your cutting is done with the left hand holding the hair, you have a fairly safe working situation. The only time you have to be concerned is when you move your thumb in and out of the thumb grip--the thumb blade might flop open if the pivot screw is too loose.

B. Extra Care Situations

When the edge hairs are cut, the scissors work close to the skin. Until you're comfortable and experienced with this kind of cutting, go slowly and always be aware of where the points of the blades are.

• When using the finger-bracing method, be sure to hold the blades at a 90 degree angle to the skin, and keep the back of the thumb blade in contact with the skin. Don't be in a hurry with this way of cutting.

•The scissors-and-comb method needs extra care because there isn't anything for the scissors to rest on while its being positioned or when cutting. Use the comb's pivot movement for extra working room with the scissors, and go slow.

•Never use scissors with the points overlapping.

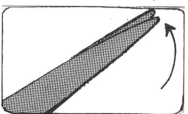

Don't use scissors with sharp points--they should always be rounded to some extent.

• Don't attempt to give a haircut to someone who can't sit still until you're an experienced haircutter. There is enough to deal with without having to dodge a person s sudden movements. (The last chapter tells how to get maximum cooperation when cutting children's hair.)

• Watch out for ears. This applies to all the edging methods, but especially the fingers-bracing method. I have only snipped a person's ear once in my haircutting career, but that was one time too many. I paid close attention to the points of the blades while edging around the ears on a short haircut--the center of the blades spoiled my day.

C. Miscellaneous Safety Tips

• Earrings. If the customer is wearing earrings that can get snagged by the comb, be sure they are taken off before you begin.

• Warts and moles. These little growths need a little extra accommodation. If a wart or mole is on the scalp, I start my bulk-removal in that area, so the comb doesn't bump into it as I'm working through the paths--it's hard to keep them in mind while striving for smooth cutting. If the growth is on the neck, it needs special handling if you shave the extra neck hairs--blot the lather off where the growth is before you begin.

•As a beginner, the way to avoid any mishap is to concentrate on what you're doing and work in a slow, deliberate manner. To this end, refrain from conversation while cutting hair; at least, keep it to a minimum. Besides the safety factor, this rule-of-thumb is important from the standpoint of quality cutting. I have had many customers who like to talk while getting their hair cut--unless I'm giving an extra easy haircut that doesn't require my concentration, I'll stop my haircutting and enjoy a good conversation. When finished, the haircutting resumes. The professionals I've worked with who were strong on chatter always produced something less than quality haircuts, and they were the ones who had problems with safety.

As far as developing tool handling skills, you now have all it takes to achieve the goal of a precision haircut. The haircut chapters show specialized uses for these skills such as sideburn trimming, tapering, and more. Before we begin our cut-by-cut how-to, you ll learn about length and shape decisions.

CHAPTER 6 THE RIGHT LENGTH

6.1 TWO PARTS TO A WELL-DONE HAIRCUT

These scissors-and-comb haircuts produce hair that not only stay in shape no matter what happens, it needs the least investment in time, money, resources, and concern. To achieve these positive results, two ingredients are essential to your success:

1. Cut the Hair Evenly. Whichever of the three haircuts you give, you will cut the hair so that it lies like shingles-on-a-roof. The tool-handling skills you've learned, and the cut-by-cut haircut chapters, assures your cutting is even and precise.

2. Cut the Hair to the Right Length. You could do an outstanding job of cutting the hair evenly, but if the hair is cut to the wrong length, it's a poor haircut. Several factors affect your decision about the right length for any person's hair:

• What is the hair type?

• What is the texture of the hair?

• What, if any, special hair problems does the person have?

• What does your customer prefer?

Consider all of these factors to figure out the best length for someone's hair. Understand that determining length is a less-than-exact science. Using the guidelines in this chapter almost always gives me excellent results on first-time haircuts, but sometimes you need to give a second, and possibly a third haircut before you have zeroed in on the very best length and cutting shape for someone's hair. Most haircut consumers know this, but it's a good idea to communicate this fact to first-time customers.

6.2 CUTTING OFF EXCESS LENGTH MAKES HAIR CAREFREE

For low-maintenance hairstyles that only need a shampoo and towel-dry every day or two, you must cut off the unnecessary hair length, and leave the hair just long enough to lie well. This rule-of-thumb applies primarily to the hair on top of the head: it is here that hair gets heavy, bulky and hard to manage. If you have a lot of hair on top, wash-and-wear haircare is difficult at best.

Your hair-length determinations are mainly concerned with the top hair. At least 90 percent of the time, sides and back hair can be cut to any length and shape-provided, of course, it blends in with the top hair. See section 6.6 for exceptions to this rule.

***

The labor movement--the folks who brought you the weekend.   Bumper sticker

6.3 THE TYPE OF HAIR MAKES A BIG DIFFERENCE

You can easily decide about length for wavy, curly, and kinky hair types because they offer complete flexibility as to length and shape. Because these hair types tend to be thick and heavy if left too long on top, most prefer a length of 1 1/2 inches or less on the top. The shorter the cutting, the straighter the hair lies; the longer the length, the curlier the hair.

Straight and slightly wavy hair tend to present problems. Cut it too short and it won't lie down; leave it too long and the hair becomes a floppy mop that can't keep a good shape. These kinds of hair are the ones that may have one or more of the special hair problems discussed later. For straighter hair, the next hair factor is the crucial one.

6.4 HAIR TEXTURE

The diameter of individual hair makes no difference on wavier, curly, or kinky hair. With straight or slightly wavy hair, this is the factor that determines the best length. The rule is: the finer the hair, the shorter it should be cut; the coarser the hair, the longer you should leave it. These general guidelines for bulk-removal length, leaves straight hair lying its best.

TEXTURE/LENGTH GUIDELINES

Fine hair	1 to 2 inches
Medium hair	1 1/2 to 2 1/2 inches
Coarse hair	2 to 3 inches or more

Most of my equal-length haircuts are 2 to 2 1/2 inches long, with about half the ear covered after the edging is done.

6.5 TEXTURE/LENGTH TEST FOR STRAIGHT HAIR

If you're unsure about the texture of the hair to be cut, use this four step test.

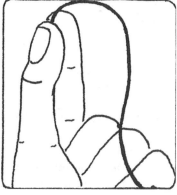 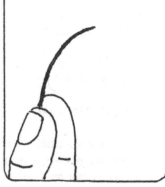

1. Pull out or cut off a top hair at the scalp. Hold the root end, and straight up.

2. Keep cutting it shorter until you have the kind of bend shown in the second drawing.

3.. Use a ruler to measure the length of the cut hair.

4. Then take a close-up look at the top hair to see at what angle the hair grows from the scalp. If the person has a fairly rare kind of hair that grows straight up (90 degrees) from the scalp, the ruler measurement is the length the top hair should be cut. If the hair

grows out at the more usual 45-degree (more or less) angle, you would subtract a half-inch from the ruler's measurement.

If the hair is thinning on top, cut it another quarter to half-inch shorter. Thinning hair tends to lie close to the head because it does not have much neighborly support. Those sparse top hairs have more fullness, if cut shorter.

6.6 SPECIAL HAIR PROBLEMS THAT AFFECT LENGTH AND SHAPE

Some heads of hair have conditions that make it necessary to cut the hair to a particular length or shape, and you might even need to limit yourself to one kind of haircut. With most people there won't be any problems, but you don't know unless you look closely at the hair. You can avoid unhappy results by doing a close inspection, and figuring these possible problems into your hair-length determinations.

A. Short Growing Hair Around the Bottom of the Sides

About 10 percent of men have this condition. No cause is known, nor can anything be done to change it. This stunted hair growth looks much like the man's beard hair. How it creeps up into the longer growing hair around the sides is not known. As a haircutter, you have to deal with it; however, it doesn't really become a problem that affects your cutting unless this condition exists more than an inch above the bottom hairline.

<u>Remedy</u> More than a question of hair length, this problem has to be dealt with in terms of which of the three layered haircuts should be given. When 1 to 2 inches of the lower hair is affected, you'll find an equal-length shaping doesn't work well. Instead of the hair lying smoothly around the edges, it wants to flip up, and the hair won't reach down to the normal length on the ears. Here is how it appears with a 2 inch equal-length cut.

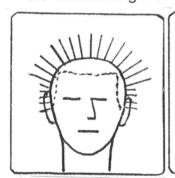
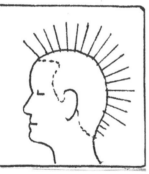
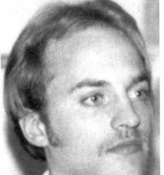
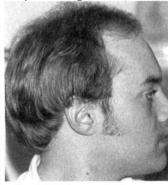

A long, layered cut covers over this problem fairly well. However, the hair doesn't even reach the bottom of the ears and it tends to flip around the edges, (but less than the equal-length cut).

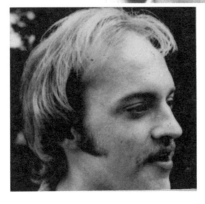
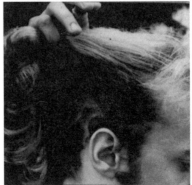

The best choice for a good fitting shape is the short, full cut. With no longer hairs covering over the short growing hairs, all the hair blend together. While this cut produces the best fit, some men don't like their hair cut this short.

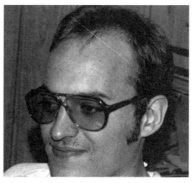
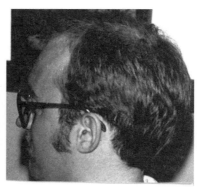

With limitations this problem presents, it's best to avoid working on someone with this condition until you've gained some experience.

B. Protruding Ears

When the tops of the ears protrude 3/4 inch or more from the head, the hair that covers them usually flips out if cut too short: it looks like wings on the sides of the head.

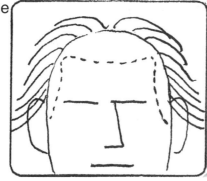

If the hairline above the ears is close to the top of the ear, the problem is worse. If there is 1/2 inch or more distance between the ear and the hairline above, the problem isn't as severe. Expect to find this condition on 5 to 10 percent of people.

Remedy Here are two good ways to deal with this problem.

• Leave the hair on the sides long enough (2 1/2 inches or more) during the bulk removal, so half or more of the ear is covered after you have done the final edging. This works well only if the texture of the hair allows that kind of longer length. If the hair has a fine texture, you are better off with the next option.

•Give an extra full, short cut with the hair cut above the ears. Extra fullness around the sides minimizes the visual effect of protruding ears, and the hair won't flip out. Because the short, full cut requires quite a bit of haircutting experience, as a beginner you should choose the first option, even if the hair is fine.

C. Double Cowlick.

Two cowlicks in the crown region likes to stand out from the head if cut too short. The area between the cowlicks is where the "rooster's tail" wants to stand on end.

Only about a quarter of double cowlicks need extra length on top to avoid hair standing on end. The difficult ones have straight, coarse-textured hair, with the two cowlicks within 1 1/2 inches of each other.

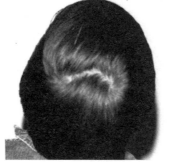
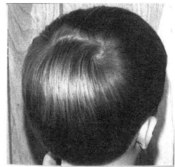

Remedy If the double cowlick is the troublesome kind, you'll need an extra inch or more of length on the upper part of the head. Use the texture/length test to help decide the length that allows the hair to lie down. Here you need to go with the length the ruler tells you--don't subtract from the measurement. I can't recall ever leaving the top hair longer than 3 1/2 inches; usually, 3 inches is plenty of length for the hair to bend into a lying position. The extra length on top may leave the bangs too long. Make your edge cuts there shorter than the normal, minimum cutting approach.

D. Low Cowlick

A cowlick in a lower-than-normal position can produce another rooster-tail condition (pages 8 and 9 in the first chapter described this stand-up problem.) The reason for this problem is quite different from a double cowlick, and the cure is exactly the opposite. This condition "pops up" in about 5 percent of the population.

Remedy To overcome the hair's battle with the forces of gravity, you need to cut the crown region short enough so the hair that wants to lie toward the top front hairline, doesn't have enough length to bend back down, toward the neck. This can be done in one of two ways on equal-length or short, full haircuts.

(1) Determine the best length for the hair, then proceed to cut the hair 1/2 to 1 inch shorter than your best guess. For example, if you decided on 2 inches, change that to 1 1/2 inches or a little shorter.

(2) After all the bulk-removal is cut to the determined length, go back to the cowlick region for some more cutting. You concentrate your re-cutting on a 3 - 4 inch wide circle with the cowlick in the center. As you work through this area, (two paths should do it,) gradually grasp the hair shorter as you approach the cowlick, and then gradually longer-to the normal length producing position-as you move away from the cowlick. This amounts to a 1/2 to 1 inch deep "sinkhole" in the haircut.

If you're giving one of the long haircuts to someone with a low cowlick, the above solutions can only be applied to the "umbrella" way of shaping, or the shorter versions of the "combination cut'. The regular version of the long, layered cut has enough length in the crown region for the hair to comfortably bend into a lying position. While the haircuts taught here normally keep a good shape for a couple of months or so, hair with a low cowlick usually needs cutting at least monthly to keep it from standing out.

E. Ducktail Neckline

Necklines that appear like a duck's tail have caused much frustration, expense, and time wasted in an effort to tame down that unruly neck hair. It doesn't lie the way they like, and as it grows longer, it starts doing flippy, contrary kinds of things.

Nothing can be done to change this condition, but we have effective ways to deal with it. This problem ranges from slight to severe.

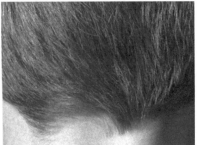
Slight

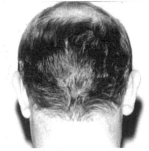
Moderate

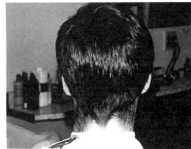
Severe

***

It's the most unhappy people who most fear change.   Mignon McLaughlin

Usually the tail is in the middle as shown above, but it can be off to one side or the other.

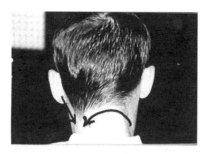

These photos all show this curvy hair grain phenomenon with short hair so it can be easily seen. Longer hair hides this condition to some extent, but long hair and a ducktail usually adds up to flippy hair at the neckline.

Remedy. In the majority of cases, the ducktail neckline does not require any special shaping or length modifications--you can cut as if it were not there. However, when moderate-to-severe ducktails combine with coarse, straight hair, you have to change your ordinary methods. Here are a couple of ways to deal with problem ducktails.
(1) Cut it extra short. An equal-length cut, with the neck-area hair tapered short, is effective, but you may need to give a short, full haircut to get it short enough. The scissors or clipper-over-comb way to taper the lower neck area maybe needed. (The beard trimming section in the last chapter shows the how-to for these cutting methods.)
(2) Leave it extra long. The long, layered cut, or the longest version of the equal-length cut, or shaping the neck hair so it has an increasing length (see the next chapter, section 5-B) leaves the hair long enough to bend over and cover this condition. While this remedy might leave the hair a little flippy at the neckline, any length between the short and long remedies has problem ducktails standing on end.
Hand combing is always a good, relaxed way to groom hair with the haircuts you are learning, but if ever a hair condition needed this hand-combed approach, it's hair with a ducktail neckline. If the rest of the head of hair has an every-hair-in-place type of grooming, the somewhat out-of-place hairs in the neck area will stand out from the rest of the hair like a sore thumb. Hand combing helps to blend all the hair together.

F. Cowlick on the Top, Front Hairline

This cowlick condition, found on 5 - 10 percent of people, normally isn't located in the hair. If you look extra close, you'll find the cowlick's center in the peach fuzz on the forehead.

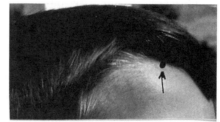

While the center of the cowlick is not in the hair, that front hairline is affected by the hair grain this cowlick establishes.
Remedy This hair-grain condition is not much of a problem as long as you *go with* the way the hair wants to lie. When you try to force the bangs to lie in a direction that is contrary to the hair's natural preferences, you need extra length on top. On some heads this kind of cowlick needs extra length even if you allow the hair to lie the way it wants. You can provide this extra length two ways:
(1) Cut the top section about one inch longer than you normally would.
(2) Leave the front 1 1/2 to 2 inches of hair--behind the top, front hairline--with a gradually increasing length. (This cutting technique is shown in the next chapter.)
One in a thousand heads of hair have a front cowlick that is a 1/2 to I inch behind the front hairline. This rare condition always needs extra length to lie well, more than what's suggested above.

6.7 THE CUSTOMER'S PREFERENCE

The last, but not least, consideration in determining the best length and shape for the hair is the customer's preference. First you must look over their hair, and then ask questions, offer suggestions, and be a real good listener. Haircut communication must be clear and concise, but of course, this is easier said than done. Ignorance, hair myths, and the wrong choice of words can muddle-up this need for clarity.
• Are they knowledgeable about hair type, texture, and special problems that may prevent many options? You may have to spend time educating beforehand.
• The bending trap. Do they want a hairstyle that requires constant bending with comb or brush, hair dryer or curling iron. hair gels or spray? Point out the hassle involved and the kind of damage that can be caused by this approach to hair, before you leave the hair with extra length so it can bend.
• Heavy hair. Many people unknowingly request to have their hair "thinned out." They don't necessarily mean they want the long, heavy top hair thinned out with thinning shears. They are just using an old term to describe their desire to get rid of the hard-to-handle hair on top. If they really want those thinners, refer to the second chapter for some education.
• Confusing terms. In my efforts to find out how a person wants their hair cut, I usually ask how they like to wear the hair around the ears (the answer to this question tells me what bulk-removal length is needed). Watch out for the term "over the ears'; for some, that means above the ears, for others, it means covering the ears. You have to take what they say, then put it into your own words and ask them if that is what they mean?
• Cutting hair from a picture. Occasionally a person brings along a picture of someone and says: I want it cut like this. Bad idea! Rarely will your customer's hair characteristics match those of the person in the picture (unless the picture is of that customer at some earlier time).. This way of expressing their haircut desires is a useful point of departure-- use the picture to explain how your wishful person's head of hair is different from the person's hair in the picture, and how that difference results in a different appearance. Lastly, point out what other options exist.
Meeting your customer's desires might require some give-and-take. With what you now know about hair versus what they desire, a little compromise may be necessary. If the customer wants you to ignore what you've learned, either do it their way or send them off to some other pro. You don't need to start your haircutting efforts with unhappy results. I don't say you'll always be right using the information in this chapter, but you'll be able to make educated judgments worth following. If your length calculations are off the mark, they won't be far off. When your best guess is a little off, that doesn't mean you have produced a poor haircut: it only means you have some room for improvement on the second cutting. Using the haircut record system described in the last chapter will help ensure you've learned from the first haircut, and improvements are made on the second.

6.8 MOST PEOPLE HAVE SPECIFIC HAIR CONCERNS

Many people have a tried-and-true knowledge about what works best on their hair. Besides smoothly cut hair that lies well and the kind of basic overall shaping given to the hair, people are concerned with particular parts of the haircut. I've arranged this list in order of importance, but it's strictly an individual matter. The last thing listed here can be your customer's big concern.

1. The Length Around the Ears. How far the hair comes down over the ear on an equal-length cut seems to be the big one for most people. Keep in mind that the length you leave the hair during bulk cutting determines the length of the hair covering the ear (see page 63). Also remember, your final edging raises the bottom edge about a half-inch or a little more, and be sure to take into account the shrinking edge-line factors explained in chapter 5, section 6.

2. Having the Hair Feather Back. Since the early 1970s, more and more people have begun wearing their hair back off the face. All three haircuts, especially the equal-length cut, can be worn this way, but it depends largely on having a Type 2 hair grain. If you have a Type 1 grain, the hair must be left at least an inch longer than normal to have it bend toward the back. Because extra length creates heavy hang-down hair, yet the extra length is needed to bend the hair, this maybe one of those patron's preferences that can't be satisfied.

3. The Bangs. Back in the 1960s and early 1970s, the length of the bangs was quite a big thing. The trend to the feathered-back approach changed this. Before, it was a matter of how much forehead showed, now the idea is to get the bangs to lie back, off to the sides or top hair. Times change, but cutting the bangs so they don't block one's vision is still a concern. Page 63 tells how the bulk-removal length determines the length of bangs.

4. Top Hair. When the top hair has too much length, it becomes heavy hair that lies flat on the head. Many people use this as their reminder that it's time for another haircut. The three basic haircuts in this book are designed for maximum body and fullness on top.

5. Neck-Hair Length. How long or short the hair is at the neckline can be a big issue.. For some it's bothersome; some have a masculine (no flips) versus feminine (hooray for flips) thing about it. The next chapter shows how to make modifications on the neck hair.

Always ask your customers what their haircut "quirks" are, and what past problems they have had with their hair and haircuts. The idea is to accommodate them whenever possible.

6.9 MY TWO HAIRSTYLING RULES

If you've ever read books or magazine articles written by well-known hairstylists, you know about the endless prescriptions for how the hair should be cut and worn--a face with prominent cheekbones needs so and so; the triangular-shaped head must have the hair cut this way; the oblong face requires more hair here, and less hair there; the round face demands..., etc. So many "experts" preach different how-tos, you'll find contradictions all over the place. I have kept my hairstyling rules simple and consistent.

I. Make the hair easy to care for and easy to ignore.
The first rule is always achievable if the person wants an unburdened head of hair. All three layered haircuts should be cut so the top hair primarily, and the rest of the hair too,

has all the excess length removed. When hair is left just long enough so it lays well--the essential hair length--you have created low-maintenance, ignorable hair.

2. Cut the hair to fit the person's size.

This rule depends on the person's hair. Some heads of hair, especially straight fine hair or hair with special problems, don't lend themselves to hair length or shape options. On the other hand, over half of the time, the heads of hair I work on allow me different choices. If the hair presents limitations, I work within those limits. If the hair gives me choices, I recommend a length and shape that balances the hair with the person's physical size. Here are some examples:

• For a tall person, cut the hair on the longer side. A shorter person would get a shorter haircut.

• For a long neck, leave the neck hair longer. A short forehead gets a shorter bulk-cutting on top, so the bangs are also shorter.

• Long sideburns fit a man with a long face, and vice versa.

This rule of fit and balance, and the above examples are not chiseled in stone. I give some haircuts where the opposite of what is suggested here works well, However, when the hair gives choices, a length and shape that's in harmony with a person's physical attributes always works well.

You now have all the ingredients it takes to get extra good results on first attempt at precision haircutting. Give yourself a few pats on the back.

***

Liberty is the only thing you cannot have unless you're willing to give it to others.
William Allen White

Next time you think you're perfect, try walking on water.
Bumper sticker

Man is the only animal that blushes, or needs to.
Mark Twain

If a man is alone in the forest and speaks, and there is no woman to hear him, is he still wrong?
Sign in a Maine diner

The man with insight enough to admit his limitations comes nearest to perfection.
Johann Von Goethe

Accomplishments will prove to be a journey, not a destination.
Dwight Eisenhower

Real happiness in life starts when you begin to cherish others.
Lama Zopa Rinpoche

Lord, help me to be the person my dog thinks I am.
Bumper sticker

A hunch is creativity trying to tell you something.
Anonymous

If you think you can or think you can't, your right.
Henry Ford

Aging gracefully requires the "pop eye" approach--I am what I am!
Unknown

CHAPTER 7 EQUAL-LENGTH HAIRCUT

7.1 INTRODUCTION

You begin by learning the haircut that proves there is **beauty in simplicity** in the endless ways of having hair cut. The uncomplicated nature of this cut makes it the easiest haircut to learn: just pull the hair out all over, and cut it to the same length. This simple way of cutting produces a shingles-on-a-roof haircut that always keeps a good shape with the least amount of haircare. These features are why this haircut's popularity goes back many generations--it has been called the layered-cut, the windblown, the afro, the feathered-cut, the radial-cut, the inch-cut, the three-inch cut, and the 90-degree haircut. Whatever its name, people love it.

The name equal-length cut implies a sameness in appearance from one haircut to the next. Don't be misled. You could give ten of these haircuts to ten people, and the final appearance of each would be quite different. The following contribute to the uniqueness:

1. Hair Factors. Hair type, hair grain, hair texture, and thickness or thinness combine to make equal-length haircuts appear different.

2. Haircut Factors. The equal-length cut lends itself to different cutting lengths: as short as one inch on finer-textured or curlier types of hair, to as long as three or more inches. In addition, this chapter teaches some easy shaping variations that leave some parts of the hair longer or shorter than the overall equal-length approach.

3. The Human Factor. Haircutting is a hand craft. When you produce things by hand, the results always vary a little from one effort to the next--it has that one-of-a-kind quality called character. These before-and-after pictures show this haircut's uniqueness:

Type 1, medium, straight hair

Type 2, medium straight hair

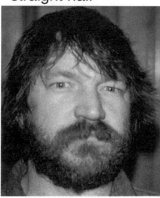

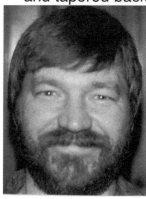

Cut to 2 inches, and tapered back

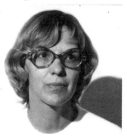

Cut to 2 1/2 inches all over

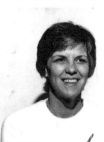

Type 2 medium
slightly wavy hair

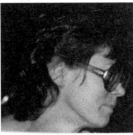

Cut to 2 inches
left longer in back

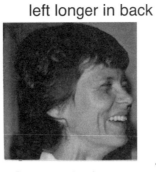

Type 2 grain.
Coarse, curly
to kinky hair

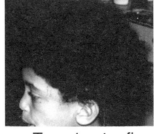

Cut to 2 inches,
back tapered

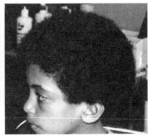

Type 1, straight
medium hair

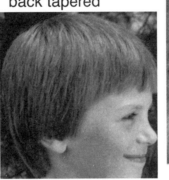

Cut to 2 inches
back tapered

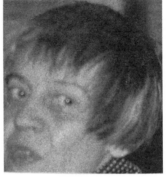

Type 1 extra fine
straight hair, low
cowlick   .

Cut to 2 inches.
cowlick area is
1 1/2 inches

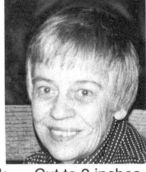

Type 1 medium
long straight hair

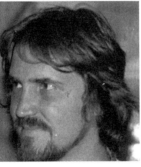

Cut to 2 1/2 inches,
bangs & neck shorter

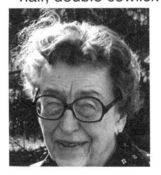

Type 2 fine wavy
hair, double cowlick

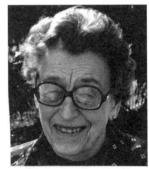

Cut to 3 inches,
sides tapered

Type 2 coarse
wavy hair

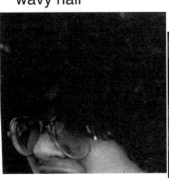

Cut to 3 inches
back tapered to

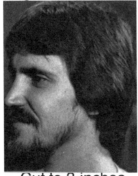

Type 2 medium
straight hair

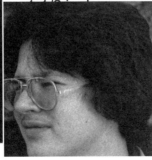

Cut to 3 inches,
back tapered to
an inch

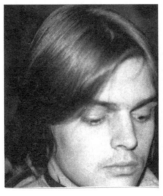

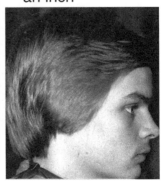

You can see there is plenty of variety in the final appearance of this haircut. As a beginner you're wondering what to expect on your first haircut? First, a warning to perfectionists: do yourself a favor and give the book to someone not burdened by faultless standards--cutting 100,000 hairs will only leave you frustrated! For those who can accept less than perfect results, I predict you'll give quality haircuts that are better than most professionals give. (This prediction comes from working with more pros than I can count, and feedback from my learners.) Here's a look at the world of professional cutters: (I) About a third of the pros do excellent work that fully meets their patron's needs. They produce precision cuts on a consistent basis. (2) Another third get "so-so" results. Sometimes it's a good cut, sometimes it's poor. They may suffer from job burn-out, or perhaps they're more interested in conversation, or in selling extra services or products. There are many things to take the mind off haircutting, but a poor haircut results when the focus drifts off. (3) The last third try to do the job, but they don't know what they are doing. These people should probably find another way to make a living. As a beginner, you have important advantages on your side:

• You care! Desire and honest effort makes a positive contribution to the results you get.
• You have 49+ years of haircutting knowledge to guide you. Many pitfalls are avoided.
• You can take whatever time is needed to do the job right--if a little change or correction is needed, you can take the time to do that.
• Your goal is healthy, easy-to-care-for hair. You could achieve an extra precise cutting on a haircut, but if the hair must have a lot of time or damaging extras in its daily maintenance, it's a sorry haircut. The haircuts you'll be giving makes it possible to practice a healthy, less-is-better way to care for hair--haircare that keeps the hair looking good with minimum effort.

Let's assume that somehow haircuts could be ranked on a 1 to 10 scale: number 1 would be a hairy disaster, and number 10 would be a perfectionist's dream. From my experience with beginners I can predict you'll start around the 7 level. With experience you'll slowly improve (with an occasional reversal) until you reach the 9 level I usually operate at. Just remember: you're not a machine that stamps out a consistent product time after time--you'll have your ups-and-downs. With the help of the haircut recording system described in the last chapter, you can improve on the haircuts that needed it.

7.2 BULK-CUTTING OVERVIEW

To go from the first to the last cut in the bulk-removal, with every hair cut to the length you want, you must use a systematic sequence of sections, pathways, and cuts. This way of cutting hair is the same approach used when mowing a lawn. You don't cut grass with a "here a cut, there a cut" approach, nor do you take a wandering path all over the lawn: to get all of the lawn cut in the most effective way, you use a systematic approach that has paths cut beside already-cut paths.

A. The Sequence to Follow

When you follow this sequence of sections, pathways, and cuts within pathways, you'll mow them off without a single "blade" being left uncut. You start on the top of the head.

***

Choose a job you love, and you will never have to work a day in your life.　　　Confucius

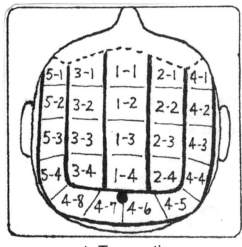

1. Top section

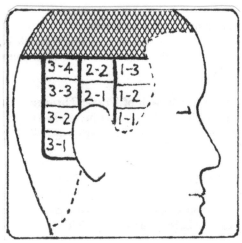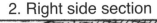

2. Right side section

The numbers represent the pathways and cuts you make. For example, 1-1 in the top section is the first pathway's initial cut. 1-2 is the second cut in the first path; 1-3 would be the first path, third cut.

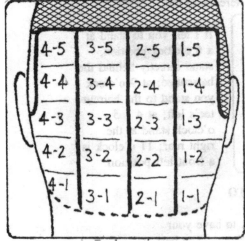

3. Back section

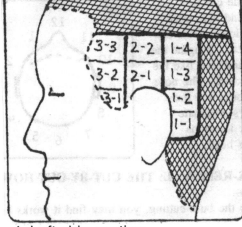

4. Left side section

Moving on, 2-1 is the second path's first cut; 2-2 is the second path's next cut; and so on. The checkered areas show the hair that has been cut as you are working around the head.

B. Why Do It This Way?

• This methodical approach means you always know where you are, where you've been, and where you're going next.

• As you move from one cut to the next, your comb travels through the hair against, or at least sideways to the hair grain. This gets the hair combed out from its lying position.

• When you work on neighboring pathways, you're able to use the guide-hair aid. While there are a few areas where you can't make use of guide-hair, over 90 percent of your cuts have this important visual help.

C. The Number of Paths and the Cuts Within a Path are Approximate

Always use the cutting sequence shown above, but keep in mind that the number of cuts in a pathway and the number of pathways in a section depend on such things as the size of the head, how thick (more cuts in a path) versus how thin (less cuts) the hair is, and the size of your hand that holds the hair. For example, I am able to use just 3 paths on the top section for some children, but, for an adult with a large head, I may have to add a couple of paths to get to the outside limits of the top section. On a smaller head, I may only need 3 cuts to get from the front to the back of the top section; a larger head could take 5 to as many as 7 cuts.

The number of pathways or cuts within a path are not important--what's important is to follow the **sequence** of sections, pathways, and cuts within the paths.

D. One Cut for Each Inch of Travel Through a Pathway

As you go through a pathway, you'll make one cut per inch of travel through the path. An average sized hand that holds the hair will make your cuts about 1 1/2 inches wide.

7.3 YOUR POSITION WHILE CUTTING

Page 56 described a couple of basic height positions that maximize your vision while cutting, and make tool handling easier. For the same reasons you also change where you stand during the haircut. To help simplify the description of where to stand while cutting the different pathways, I refer to the hours of the clock.

Stand behind the customer and look down at the top of their head. Imagine the head is numbered like the face of a clock. The nose is 12 o'clock, and the other hours designate your other locations around the head.

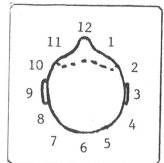

If I tell you to stand at a 6 o'clock position, stand directly behind the person; at 9 o'clock you stand to the patron's left; at 4 - 5 o'clock stand at the right rear; 11 o'clock is a front left position.

Before starting, go back to chapter 3, and be sure you've followed the steps in "Preparations for Haircutting Success". Do the approximate cutting (chapter 4) if needed, and you're ready to begin the bulk-removal cutting!

7.4 THE CUTTING BEGINS

A. Top Section

Begin with the first pathway. Move from the front-top-center hairline straight back to the top center of the crown region. The 1 1/2 inch width of the path, and the one cut for each inch of travel back to the crown region is easy to work with; however, the width can be narrower or wider, depending on the size of your left hand. You may feel more comfortable using a couple of shorter cuts rather than one closing of the scissors for each cutting step shown.

Don't try to get too much hair between those holding fingers. Holding too much hair causes the kind of unevenness shown at the right. Thicker heads of hair are affected more by this overloading the hand problem.

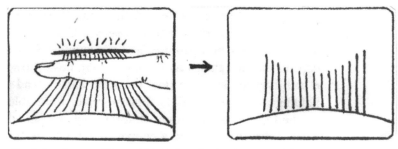

To get started, stand behind in a 6 o'clock position. Wet the hair thoroughly and comb it forward on top and down the sides and back. Rewet the hair as often as necessary during the haircut. If needed, use the helping-hand method (page 54) to get the hair combed up for the first cut.

Pathway 1 You may need to make more than 4 cuts on a large head or thick hair. When you reach the top back of the head, comb the top hair forward again and go back through path 1 a second time. (You may not cut off any hair, but you're sure this important first path is cut to the desired length, and it's a straight path

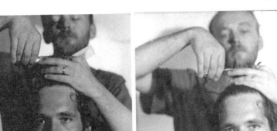

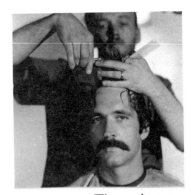

Path 1, cuts 1 through 4

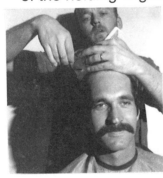 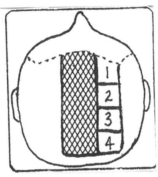 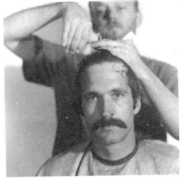

There is no guide hair to use on this first path--be extra sure the holding hand produces a consistent length.

Pathway 2 In path 2 you use the important guide hair aid. Be sure to comb up some of that already-cut hair from path I as you work through path 2. On this first photo, the scissors point to the guide hair at the "V" of the holding fingers.

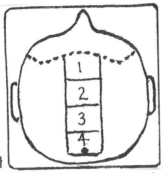

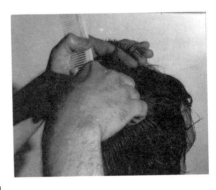

Path 2, cuts 1 through 4

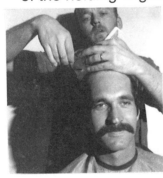 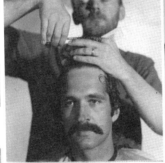 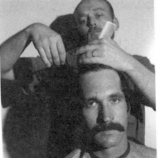 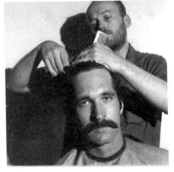

Remember to re-comb the hair forward on top, after you finished each path on the top section. The helping-hand aid is used before the first cut on all the pathways you make. Continue at the 6 o'clock position. Remember to keep a pinching pressure between the holding fingers until the comb is reinserted in the hair after each cut is made in the path.

The guide-hair at the "V" of your holding fingers does not show in these photos, but it was there after careful combing and positioning of the holding hand.

Pathway 3

This path requires the same 6 o'clock position. Now the guide hair shows at the tips of the holding fingers. Don't cut those guide hairs, just use them.

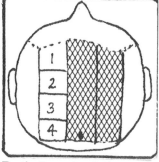 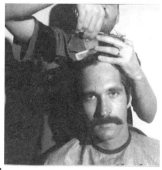

Path 3, cuts 1 through 4

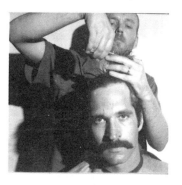 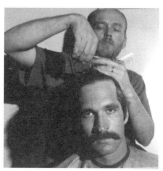 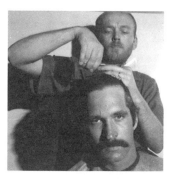

Pathway 4

This pathway is the longest (most cuts in a path) of all the paths. Start in at the front, just below pathway 2. Path 4 goes along the upper right side and then back around the upper back part of the head where it meets the back part of paths I, 2 and 3.

The first 4 or 5 cuts are done while in a 5 o'clock position. As you work your way around the back of the head to the last cut, change your position a little with each cut until you're in a 8 or 9 o'clock position.

Assuming an average shaped head, this path goes along one of the major curves of the head. Either the holding fingers conform to this curved shape, or an extra path is needed between this path and the second path. This overlapping path is done after you've made the cuts in this fourth path (pages 53 described this in more detail).

The guide-hair is at the "V" of the holding fingers. It may take as many as 9 or 10 cuts, or as few as 5, to reach the left rear corner.

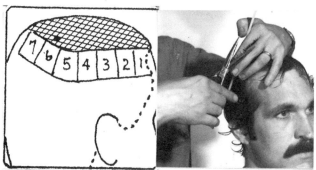 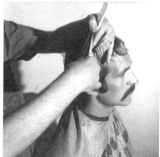 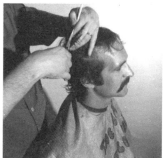

Path 4, cuts 1 through 7

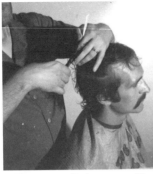
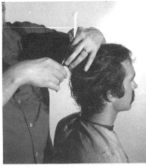
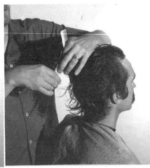
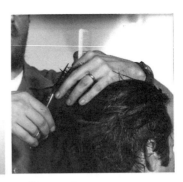

The cowlick area "behaves" itself if the hair is allowed to lie the way it wants.

Pathway 5 For me, the easiest way to handle this pathway is to stand at the 10 - 11 o'clock position and use the comb-away hand-tool manipulation. You can use the basic manipulation at 6 - 7 o'clock, but to me it feels awkward with my arm held high. The comb-away approach has the guide hair at the "V" of the holding fingers.

The comb-away requires you to be extra aware when the left hand is positioned. There is a tendency to have the holding fingertips a bit closer to the scalp than the length at the "V"--keep this in mind and guard against it. Also, the comb-away has the points of the blades moving toward the face--go slow and know where the points of the scissors are at all times . Path 5 is another curved area, handle it as you did path 4.

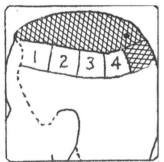
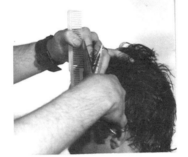
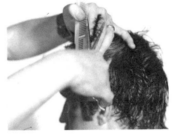

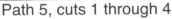

Path 5, cuts 1 through 4

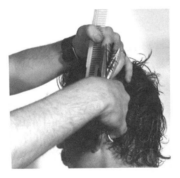
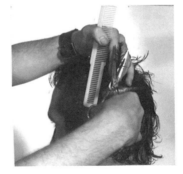

Now that you have the top section done, it's time to start working on the side hair.

B. Right Side Section

For the sides and back sections, position your chair as low as possible for the best line of vision and tool handling ease. When you cut around the sides and back the guide-hair shows at the "V" of your holding fingers. You'll always have guide-hair to use except for:the first path on the right side and the area behind the right ear, down to the bottom of the back. Just a few cuts with no neighboring cuts to rely on--go slow on these cuts, and be sure your hair holding hand is in its length-producing "groove".

Pathway 1 Stand at a 7 to 9 o'clock position with the patron helping by bending his or her head toward you. Always comb the hair straight down on the sides and back before starting out on any of the pathways. Usually you'll make 2--3 cuts in this pathway, but make as many cuts as needed to get up to the cut hairs on the top section. As with the first path on the top section, go through this beginning pathway twice to be sure it's cut evenly. Because of the irregular shape of the temple's hairline, some of your cuts going up this first pathway will have you hold and cut small amounts
of hair. What you want with this first path is get it relatively straight so the next couple of paths can also be straight. These in-line pathway routes are easier to handle than twisted ones that follow the hairline.

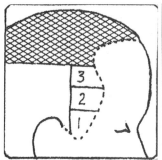 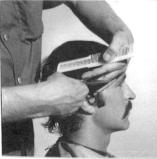 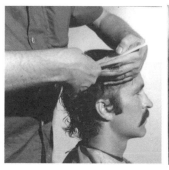 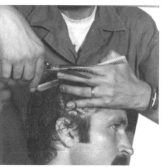

Path 1, cuts 1 through 3

Pathway 2 This path is directly above the ear and you need to take care when starting your comb-out so you don't snag the top of the ear with the comb. Use the sideways comb trick (page 55) or the helping-hand method, Stay in the 7 to 9 o'clock position.

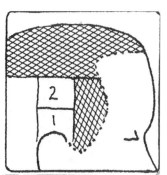 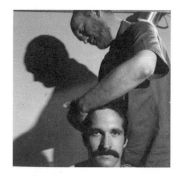 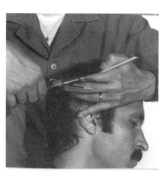

This path may need 3 cuts, but usually a couple are all it takes.

Path 2, cuts 1 - 2

Pathway 3 The last pathway on the right section starts behind the ear, at about mid-ear level. The first cut won't have any guide-hair to use, but the rest of the cuts have it. Stand at a 7 - 8 o'clock position.This pathway maybe on one of the major curve areas of the head. If the head curves, have your holding fingers conform to the curve, or use the straight approach with an extra pathway between this path and the next one.

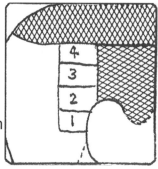

Path 3, cuts 1 - 4

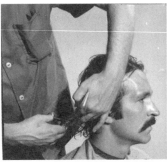
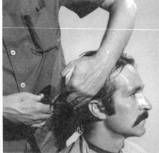
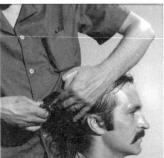
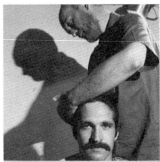

C. Back Section

The back hair can have some changes from the all-the-same-length cutting you've been striving for. Besides an equal-length cutting on the back, you can taper the bottom hair shorter or it can be left longer. If you want to modify your equal-length cutting, skip ahead now to page 102

Back to equal-length cutting. Pathway 1 on the back section is usually on another major curve--have your cutting conform to it. Stand at the 7 or 8 o'clock position for the first pathway. For each succeeding pathway, move toward the front left side until you're at the 10 or 11 o'clock position for the last pathway in this section.

Pathway 1 As usual, start by combing the hair down. It may take 6 or 7 cuts to work your way up to the top section. One cut per inch gets you there. The first 2 or 3 cuts in this path are below path 3 on the right side section--no guide hair to use here.

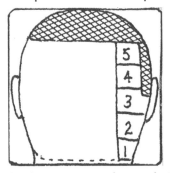
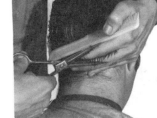
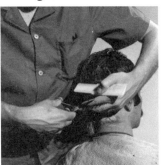

Path 1, cuts 1 through 5

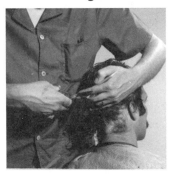
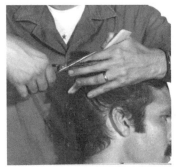
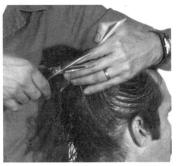

Pathway 2 Guide-hair is at the "V" of the holding fingers for all remaining cuts in the bulk cutting. A small head may only need 4 cuts going up the back, and you may get by with only 3 paths. ***

Quality is never an accident; it is always the result of high intention, sincere effort, intelligent direction and skillful execution.

Will A. Foster

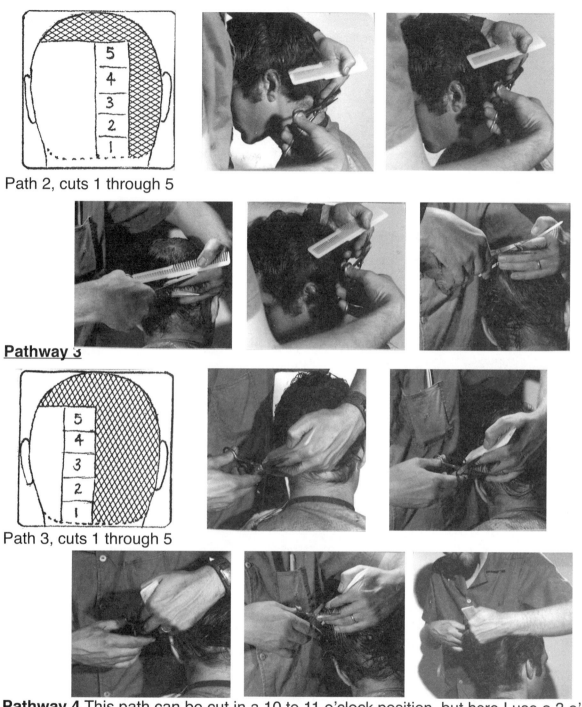

Path 2, cuts 1 through 5

Pathway 3

Path 3, cuts 1 through 5

Pathway 4 This path can be cut in a 10 to 11 o'clock position, but here I use a 3 o'clock. Keep in mind this is probably on a curved area--have the holding hand conform to it.

***

Politics is about the improvement of people's lives.   Senator Paul Wellstone

Our ideals, laws and customs should be based on the proposition that each generation in turn becomes the custodian rather than the absolute owner of our resources--and each generation has the obligation to pass that inheritance on to the future.   Alden Whitman

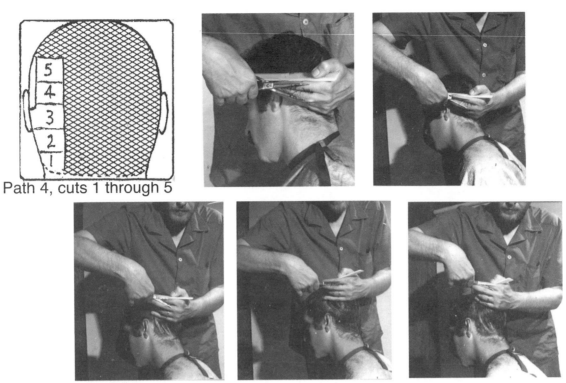

Path 4, cuts 1 through 5

D. Left Side Section

Pathway 1 Now get into the 3 - 4 o'clock position for this cutting. About 4 cuts will do it.

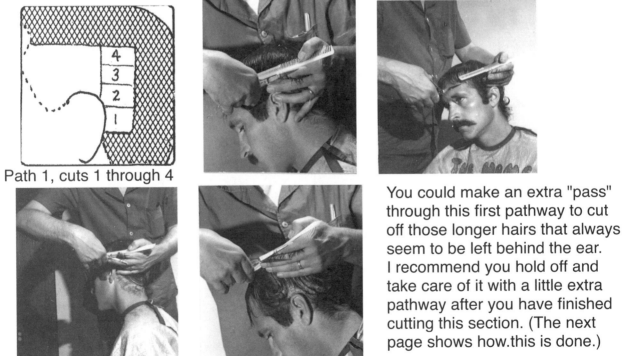

Path 1, cuts 1 through 4

You could make an extra "pass" through this first pathway to cut off those longer hairs that always seem to be left behind the ear. I recommend you hold off and take care of it with a little extra pathway after you have finished cutting this section. (The next page shows how.this is done.)

Pathway 2 Here again, use whatever means are necessary to start out without snagging the top of the ear with the comb.

***

Be the change you seek in this world.   Mohatmas Gandhi

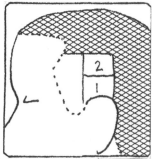

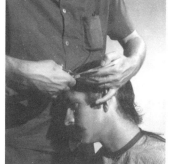

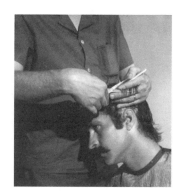

Path 2, 2 or 3 cuts

Pathway 3 This is probably the last path to cut.

On the other hand, if the hair grows far onto the temple region, you may have to make one extra path to finish the left side section.

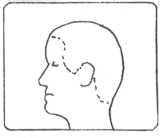

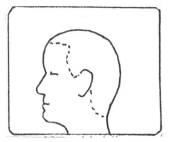

Unusual hairline

Normal hairline

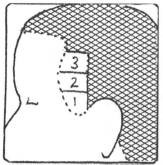

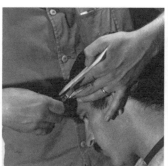

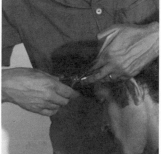

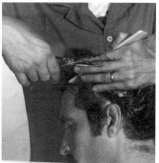

Path 3, cuts 1 through 3

If the left side needs the extra path at the front of this section, do it now. Before finishing with the bulk-removal, just a bit more cutting is needed behind the left ear. For some reason, that area behind the ear doesn't get cut as evenly as the rest. To remedy this, move to a 11 o'clock position for this remedial cutting. This may look awkward, but I've found it's the most effective way to smooth off this area.

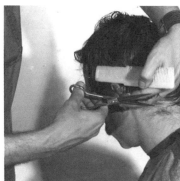

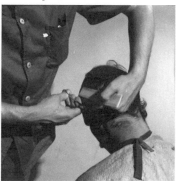

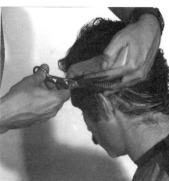

While you're at it, take an 8 o'clock position and check for longer hairs behind the right ear.

If the back-bottom area hair isn't going to be tapered, you have now finished the first-time-through bulk-removal cutting.

7.5 TWO APPROACHES TO CUTTING NECK HAIR

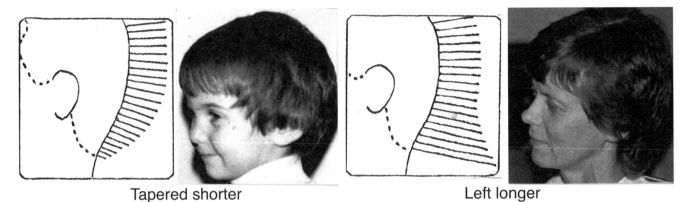

Tapered shorter   Left longer

A. 2-Step Tapering

If the back-bottom hair is to be tapered, making it shorter than the rest of the hair, now is the time to do it.

For purposes of illustration, say you have given a 3 inch equal-length cut, with 3 inches of hair hanging below the neck's hair-line.

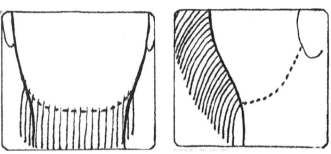

Step 1 Using the finger-bracing-the-scissors or pull-and-cut method, cut off 1 1/2 to 2 inches. Leave 1 to I 1/2 inches of hair below the hairline. Round the corners a bit.

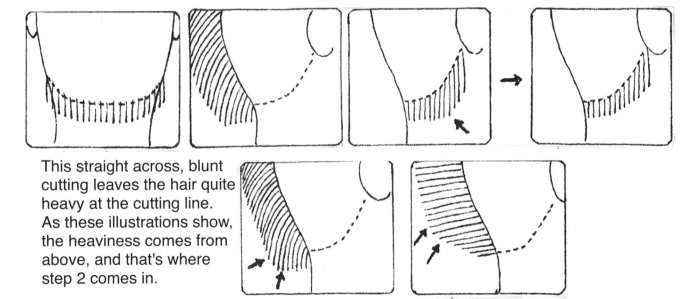

This straight across, blunt cutting leaves the hair quite heavy at the cutting line. As these illustrations show, the heaviness comes from above, and that's where step 2 comes in.

Step 2 If you were to stop after the first step, the hair would appear as if it had been given a "bowl-cut', and it would tend to flip out and be shaggy around the bottom.

To get this hair to lie well, you need to concentrate your next cutting (tapering) efforts 1 or 2 inches above the edge hair. The kind of smoothness shown in the illustration at the right is the goal.

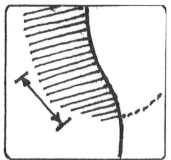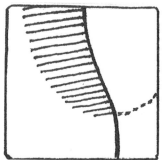

To smooth off this uneven hair, switch to a diagonal positioning with your left hand's, fingertips touching, or almost touching the neck. This diagonal position has the holding fingers curve away from the neck.

If the holding fingers were in a vertical position, the neck would be in the way. Bent scissors would be needed to cut the held hair--that neck gets in the way.

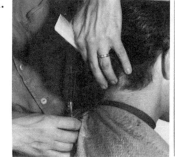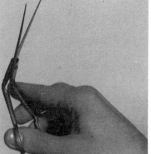

To begin, stand at a 7 o'clock position. Have the head bent down as far as possible. When you've worked over to the left side (one cut per inch of travel across the bottom), you'll stand at a 9 or 10 o'clock.

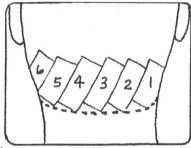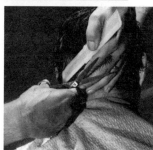

As you can see above, here we begin to cut back on the use of photos; this will be the case until we get to the edging part of the haircut.

When your left hand is positioned, you want to have guide-hair showing at the fingertips and the "V' of the holding fingers. If the hair has been left longer than a couple of inches, your hand may need to be positioned at some distance from the scalp. Just cut the longer hair between the two guide hair aids to get this hair smoothed off.

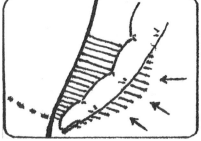

After finishing this path, make one more path across the back, just above the previous one to check for smoothness. Here a vertical position can be used because the neck won't be in your way. Trim as needed while using guide-hair at the fingertips (from the previous path) and at the "V" (the already-cut hair from the first-time-through cutting). If the hair you're working on has a ducktail neckline, you may have to use the comb-away method for the bottom, right side neck hair (see page 145 for more on this.)

Another Approach. While I recommend this 2-step method of tapering neck hair for beginners (it can also be used on other tapered cutting,) it's not my preferred method on the neck area. I get the same results, but much quicker, by using a stepping-out method on the first-time-through bulk-removal. With this approach I increase the length I leave the hair with each manipulation made while going up a pathway on the back of the head. Repeating the same stepping-out cuts on each pathway in the back, gets the hair fairly well tapered, ready for a little smoothing off on the second-time-through cutting. How many stepping-out cuts are made and what length to leave them are questions that depend on the overall length of the rest of the hair, and on what the person likes. These examples are fairly typical.

On a 2 1/2 inch equal-length cut, the first cut at the neck leaves the hair 1 1/2 inches long. Move up an inch for the next cut in the path, and here it's left 2 inches. Another inch up and you're at the 2 1/2 inch cutting you've given to all the hair. If your equal-length cutting left the hair 3 inches, the cuts would be 1 1/2, 2, and 2 1/2 inches before you're up to the 3 inch length given to the rest of the hair.

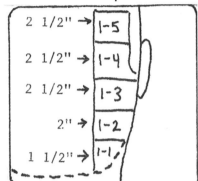

After the first path is cut, repeat the same length producing cuts on each of the back's pathways. Guide-hair is used after the first path is cut.

I don't recommend this way of tapering hair for the beginner because I feel it requires a level of skill that maybe too difficult for some. If you think you can do it, go ahead and use it--but in time you ought to be able to handle this faster (and easier) way of tapering.

B. **Longer Shaping for Neck Hair**

To achieve a gradually longer length to the back hairs, comb the hair at the bottom of the neck up, and make the first cut in the pathway higher up than you do for equal-length cutting.

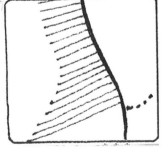

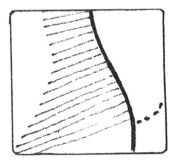

Position for Longer Shaping   Equal-length Position

With the hair below your left hand combed up farther, while held at the same length-producing position used on the rest of the bulk-removal cuts, that bottom hair is left gradually longer.

For example, if your hand is positioned 2 inches up from the hairline, the hair is left with this extra length:

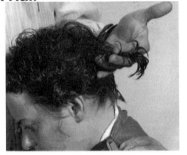

The higher up the first cut is made, the longer the hair is left. If the first cut is 3 inches up, this would result:

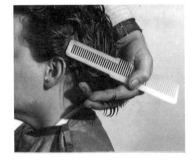

***

It's not that I'm so smart, it's just that I stay with problems longer.   Albert Einstein

On the other hand, the lower the first cut is made, the less extra length will be left. If the first cut is I inch up from the bottom hairline, this would be the result:

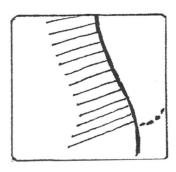

Whatever height is choosen, you'll repeat it with the first cut on each of the pathways in the back section. The usual starting point is 2 to 2 1/2 inches up for those who like the extra length.

This gradually longer length way to cut can also be done to the bangs. If you had a front hairline cowlick needing a longer length in order to lie well, you comb the hair back and hold it behind the front hairline--the first cut is made there while using the same length-producing position used on the rest of the cuts in the path.

You hold and cut behind the front hairline instead of in the normal, straight-out-from-the-head position, right at the hairline.

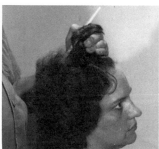 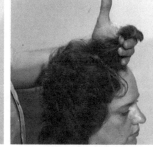

Behind hairline   At hairline

To do this type of shaping, whether it is neck hair or the bangs, the hair at the hairline has to be long enough to reach back, and then up to the holding fingers.

7.6 GET IT ALL SMOOTHED OFF

Now the unevenness that's left from the bulk-cutting is cut. This procedure has two parts to it.

A. Correcting Major Length Differences

Here you are concerned with the hair on one side of the head being left longer than the hair on the other side, or with one side of a section left longer than the other. When you cut hair with your hand holding the hair, it's very difficult to get an area cut shorter than the rest. However, it is fairly easy for beginners to leave the hair longer, especially by the time the left side section is cut.

To check the hair's length, pull the hair out in 10 - 12 locations and measure it with a ruler. Differences in length of more than 1/2 inch should be recut as needed.

• If you find a large area of 10 or more square inches, go to an area that is cut to the correct length and check your holding hand position there when the hair is held out from the head. Go back to the longer area and use the same hand position for the recutting.

• A small area is done by combing out neighboring, correctly-cut hair and using it as guide-hair while recutting the longer hair. Rarely (if ever) will you find an area that has been cut too short, but, if you should happen to discover this, you have two options:

(1) Leave it be. For the beginner, I recommend that you accept your boo-boo. Before you give your next haircut, take the time to practice the left/holding hand exercises until you can do them blindfolded.

(2) If the hair can be cut shorter, go back over all the bulk-removal and get the rest of the hair cut as short as your short spot.

If the ruler shows less than 1/2 inch differences in length, they are taken care of with the next part of the smooth off process.

B. Minor Length Differences: The Second-Time-Through Cutting

This "polishing" part of the haircut has just a few photos to show the sequence to use and the position you'll be in. The hair you cut off here may not fill a thimble--that is usually enough to make the difference between a good haircut and an extra good one. During the second-time-through use the same hair length-producing position with your holding hand as used on the first-time-through bulk-removal; however, now your hand is held in a different direction. This change in holding direction reveals the longer than normal culprits that need cutting. As it was with bulk-cutting, you work your way through pathways with the cuts about 1 1/2 inches wide, and you make one cut for each inch of travel through the path. The rule for this second cutting is: cut only if needed.

As you go through the entire head of hair, checking for unevenness, many times the hair you hold out from the head doesn't need cutting: good for you--leave it be.

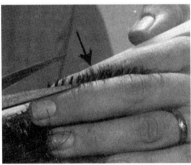

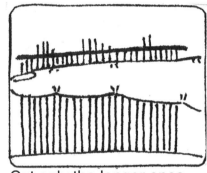

Leave well-enough alone   Cut only the longer ones

I usually ignore unevenness of 1/8 inch or less (the arrow in the photo above points to such a glitch). Yes, this book is about precision haircutting, but if I were to fret about 1/8 inch differences in length, I'd be getting too close to perfectionist haircutting. Whether the uneven hairs you cut are 1/100 or 1/2 inch longer than the rest, be sure that you only cut the longer hairs while using the shorter hairs as a guide--don't cut them. This is the systematic sequence of cuts that gets all the hair checked over and cut as needed.

1.Top Section. The hair is divided into 2 halves.

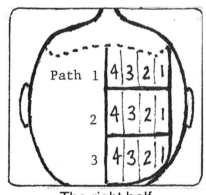

The right half

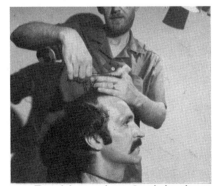

Positioned at 9 o'clock

On this right section, the holding fingers point toward the crown. The holding fingers point toward the front on the left section.

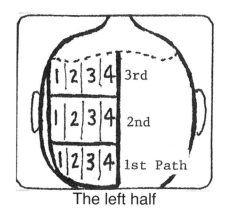

The left half

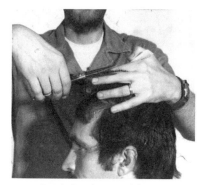

3 o'clock position

Always comb
the hair away
from you
before
making your
cuts through
the pathway.

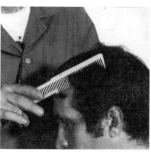

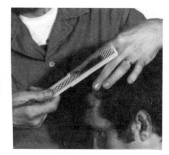

Have the chair in a higher
position for this cutting--the
same as was used for bulk-
cutting on the top section.
Keep this higher position
for all remaining second-
time through cutting.

2. Right Side Section.

Here the holding
fingers point to the
bottom hairline. This
is the way it will be
for all the remaining
second-time-through
cutting.

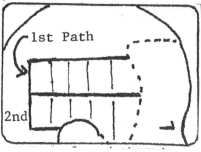

4 - 5 cuts in the path

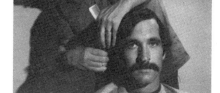

5 o'clock position

The sequence of cuts is not shown in the diagram above because the sequence used depends on the grain of the hair. If you're working on a Type 1 grain, comb the hair to the front, then make 4 to 5 cuts from the front to the back of this section. If the hair has a Type 2 grain, comb the hair toward the back of the head. Begin at the back of the section as you use the comb-away method to work forward to the front hairline.

3. Back Section.

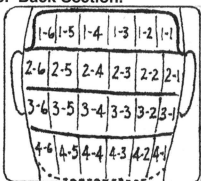

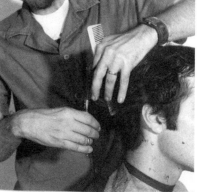

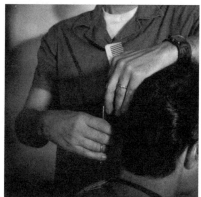

Depending on head size and the size of your left hand, you may have as few as 3

paths, or as many as 5. Position yourself at about 7 o'clock and then move to 9 or 10 o'clock as you get to the end of each pathway. Return to 7 o'clock for the next, lower pathway.

If the hair has a strong ducktail neckline hair grain, the bottom 1 or 2 paths may need the comb-away manipulation on the right side of the neck. Start at the center of the tail and cut toward the right side of the neck; back to the tail, then over to the left side using the basic manipulation.

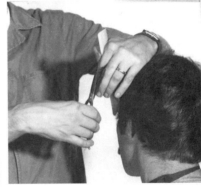

Note, if the bottom neck hair has been tapered shorter by using the beginner's 2-step method, the second-time-through cutting on the lower back has already smoothed-off. However, If you see some unevenness, go over it again. If the stepping-out method was used, the hair needs a second-time-through cutting now--use the diagonal hand positioning for the path across the bottom. If you modified your equal-length cutting so the hair is left longer at the bottom of the neck, there is no way to do this smooth-off cutting with your holding hand held in a vertical direction--the only way to deal with this gradually increasing length is to repeat the same cutting procedure used to get the increasing length during the first-time-through. As with all your second-time-through cutting, you may not have to shorten a single hair, but checking insures that it's cut right.

4 Left Side Section.

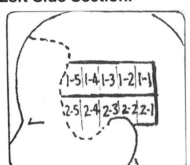
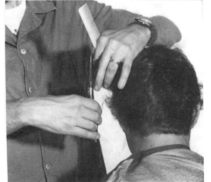
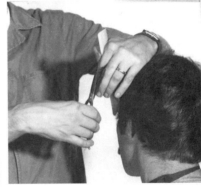

In this last section, you cut 2 paths as you did on the right side. Start out in a 9 or 10 o'clock position and move to 11 o'clock as you get to the end of the pathways. You could reverse the sequence of cuts and use the comb-away method if the hair has a Type 1 grain, but the sequence shown normally works well with Type 1 and Type 2 hair grains when the basic hand-tool manipulation is used. This is about the time I get feelings of accomplishment--the hair is shaped-up, and there is just a little more to do.

7.7 EDGE-CUTTING

This part of the haircut process is similar to the second-time-through cutting in that very little hair needs to be cut. With the exception of the edging to the hair covering the ears and possibly the lower temple area hair, all you do is cut as little as possible.

The sequence of cuts used here makes it possible to rely on guide-hair for nearly all the cuts (exceptions are pointed out). The idea is to use a bit of the already-cut, neighboring hair as a guide for the next cut you make, whenever possible.

Keep in mind that you want your edge-line cutting to conform to and be equal distance from the hairline. While there are some exceptions to this rule that will be explained with the step-by-step photos, even the exceptions require you to be aware of the shape of the hairline. To be aware, comb the hair back or up and away from its lying position so the hairline can be seen. When you comb the hair back to the cutting position, keep a mental picture of the hairline to which your cutting conforms.

A.**Bangs.** Start on the left side of the bangs while standing at 3 or 4 o'clock. 3 or 4 cuts using the modified-bulk removal edging method will get you over to the right side.

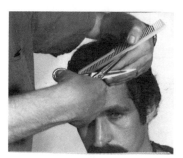 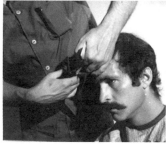 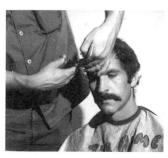

After the first cut, be sure to comb up a little of the cut hair to use as guide hair for each new cut you make.

Due to the 2 inch length the hair was left during the bulk-removal, the left hand has a fanned-out position. If it had been left longer (2 1/2 or more inches), the spacer fingers would be tucked up under the held hair. The pull-and-cut method is a good alternative to this method--this approach requires 11, 12, and I o'clock positions.

After you've finished this cutting, move to a 1 o'clock position and comb the hair forward onto the forehead. Use the finger-bracing-the-scissors method to cut any stragglers.

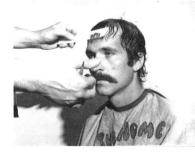 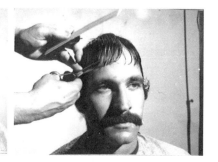

Be sure you don't cut any of the temple region hair when cutting the bangs. Comb the side hair toward the back of the head, so it's out of your way.

It's usually best if the bottom of the bangs are cut so they are equal distance from the front hairline, even if the bangs are to be worn so they lie off to one side. This way of cutting insures the bangs stay in good shape no matter which way they end up lying.

B. Temple Region-Right Side.

For our purposes, this part of the edging is divided into two parts. While the hairline in this region can take a variety of shapes, what's shown here is fairly common.

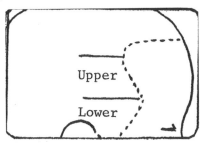

Upper

Lower

***

How long is a minute? It depends on which side of the bathroom door you're on.

Anonymous

1. **Upper part.** If the hair I'm cutting has the more common hairline shape, and if the hair is straight or wavy, I won't do any edging on the upper part--the hair always lies down (Type 1 hair grain) or toward the back of the head (Type 2 hair grain), so with no hair lying out on the edges, I just leave it be.

I do the edging on the upper part only if I'm working on curlier hair, or if the hair has one of these less common hairlines in the temple region, plus a Type 1 hair grain.

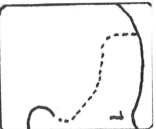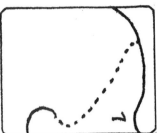

This upper temple area is easily cut by using the pull-and-cut method with you in a 12 or 1 o'clock position. As with the bangs, your cutting here will be minimal--just a little trimming does it. Avoid cutting the bangs by combing them away before you begin.
2. **Lower part**. The lower portion, unlike the upper part, always needs a little edging and sometimes more than just a little. If you've given a longer version of the equal-length cut, most folks, especially those with the straighter hair, need to have this hair cut short enough so it won't end up in the eyes if windblown. Curlier hair usually isn't affected by this problem because of its springy growth: a minimum cutting works well on curls.

If the hair is long enough, you could use the pull-and-cut method, standing at the 1 - 2 o'clock position. A couple of cuts ought to take care of it. (Note my method of cutting: be sure your cutting is done on the inside of the holding fingers, not above them as shown.)

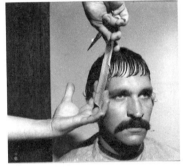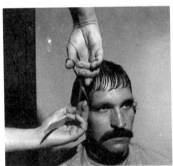

With shorter hair, the finger-bracing method works well, but if the hair wants to lie toward the back of the head, the scissors-and-comb method is needed.

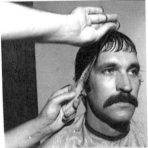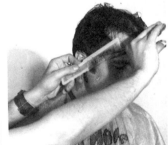

You always want the cutting line to be parallel to (equal distance from) the lower temple's hairline.

3. **Right Sideburn**. If the customer doesn't have sideburns, skip ahead to the next edging step. Before cutting, get the longer side hair above the burns out of the way. Comb the side hair as shown here--this gets the hair tucked-in behind the ear.

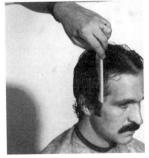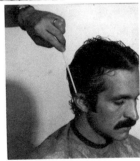

Comb the sideburn hair toward the ear. Use the finger-bracing-the-scissors method to cut the hair close to the sideburn's back hairline. Then comb the hair toward the face and cut in front of the sideburn:

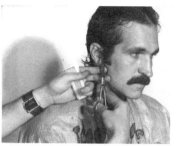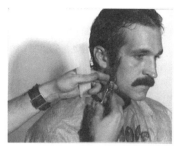

Curlier hair needs the scissors-and-comb edging method on the burns. However, now the comb is held *perpendicular* to the skin rather than lying flat on the skin.

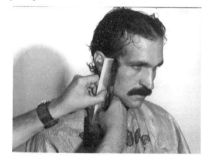

Position the comb, then move it forward to the hairline. Stop the comb before it's out of the hair, and make the cut.

This approach is used on the back of the sideburn, but now the comb is held above the sideburn. Insert the comb in the middle of the sideburn and move it toward the back edge--the cut is made with the comb still in the hair.

The scissors-and-comb method used on the backside of the burns needs this position for the comb. This upside-down approach is done with the teeth at the end of the comb. Hold the rest of the comb away from the scalp so you avoid combing into the hair above the burns.

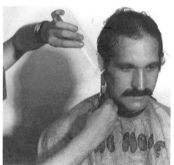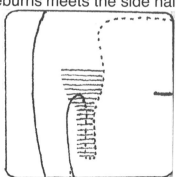

Either way of trimming sideburns works well for straight or wavy hair. However, curlier hair maybe left with the burns too bushy. Skip ahead to beard trimming in the last chapter--the scissors-over-comb method shown there will "whittle down" those burns. After the sideburns are trimmed, the length of the sideburn hair will be as short as 1/4 inch (scissor-over-comb cutting) to as long as 1/2 inch or a little more (finger-bracing cutting on the sideburn's edges). If the bulk-removal length on the side hair is 1 1/2 inches long or longer, a length difference will exist where sideburns meets the side hair.

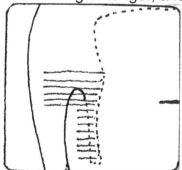

If the side hair is 1 1/2 inches or less, the side hair gets tapered and blends with the shorter side-burn hair when the lower temple and around the ear edging is done. If more tapering is needed, do it with the finishing touches.

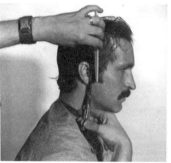

***

The best and least expensive way to improve your looks is with a smile.　　Anonymous

If the bottom of the sideburns need to be raised, just comb the hair down and use the finger-bracing method with short snips. Move forward 1/8 to 1/4 inch after you make a cut and reopen the scissor blades. This cut-open-move approach leaves a line across the burns that makes it easy to shave the hair left below the line.

How long to leave sideburns is a question without an easy answer. Whatever the person prefers is the obvious choice. For myself, I like to see some sideburn showing beneath the side hair.

Trimming sideburns, and the rest of the edging around the sides and back, is best done in a position that has your eyes on the same level as the cutting you do.

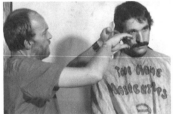
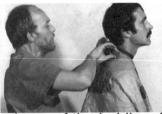

4. Right Side Hair. You cut straight across here, ignoring the shape of the hairline. How much hair you leave covering the ear was dealt with back on page 63.

First, comb the hair above the ear and in front of the ear forward like this:

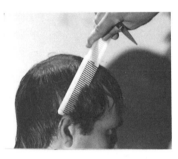
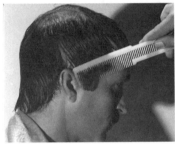
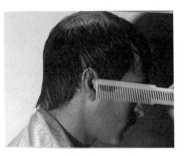

This gets the hair that tends to lie toward the back of the head (above the ears) cut off in front of the ears. They won't appear in front of the ear later, making a ragged edge-line.

Then, comb all the side hair, from the temple hairline to the back of the ear, straight down. Use the pull-and-cut method with the cutting done on the inside of the holding hand. Start at the face side and cut to the the back edge of the ear; this takes about 2 to 3 manipulations.

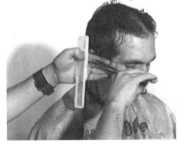
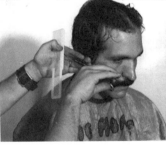

After cutting a straight line to the back edge of the ear, use the scissor-and-comb or pull-and-cut methods to round off the corner where the lower temple hair meets the side edging.

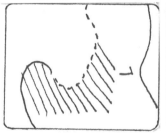
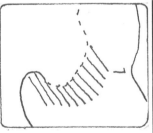
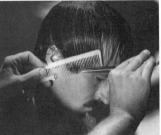
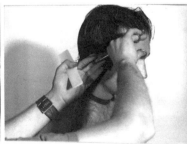

5. Right Side of the Neck. Before we begin this edging, you need to know how the different approaches to cutting the lower neck hair (during the bulk-removal) affects the edge line you cut.

1) If you gave an equal-length cutting, your edging line follows this kind of path.

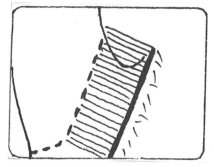 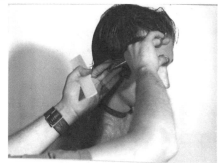

(2) If you tapered-in the back bottom hair, the edge-cutting takes this kind of shape.

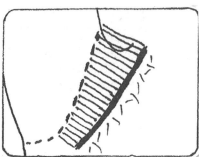 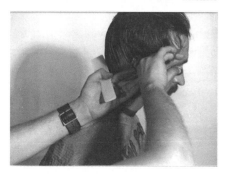

If the hair toward the bottom is too short to use the pull-and-cut, use the finger-bracing or scissors-and-comb methods on the shorter portion.

(3) The long cutting approach dictates this kind of edge-cutting line.

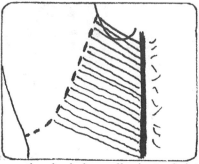 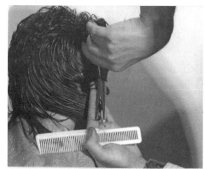

Note that in each case, the hair is pulled straight away from the hairline, and the cutting occurs as close to the skin as possible. With this edging, return to a minimum cutting. Cutting the side of the neck edge-line, starts where your covering the ear cuts left off. Use that cut hair at the back edge of the ear as guide-hair for your first pull-and-cut. The guide-hair appears (with careful combing) at your finger tips. It takes 2 to 3 pull-and-cuts to get down to the bottom.

6. Bottom Neckline. Cut the edge-line straight across. The edging method to use depends on how you shaped the lower neck hair during the bulk-removal.

(1) If you gave a long cutting use the modified-bulk-removal or the pull-and-cut.Going from right to left will take 3 to 4 manipulations with either method.

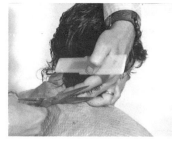

***

If you can smile when everything is going wrong, you're either a nitwit or a repairman.

Anonymous

(2) Equal-length cutting in the back lends itself to the pull-and-cut, followed by the finger-bracing approach for left-over stragglers.

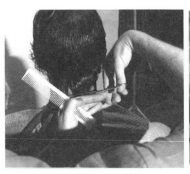 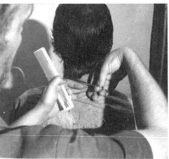 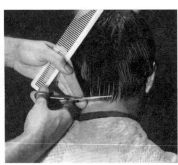

Don't follow my example in the first two photos-- do your cutting on the inside of the holding fingers.

(3)The shorter, tapered bulk-cutting usually leaves the bottom hair too short for the pull-and-cut, so use the finger-bracing-the-scissors or the scissors-and-comb method. Start at the right corner and proceed to the left. If you're working on a ducktail neckline, start at the tail and work your way to the right edge-back to the tail and then to the left side.

After you've snipped your way to the left corner, go to the right corner, and round off the area where the two straight edge-lines meet.

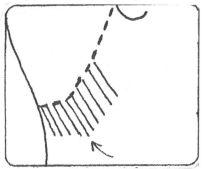 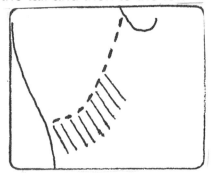

If the customer has a ducktail, inform them about the nature of this hair grain condition, and why your straight-across cutting line never stays that way. As soon as they bend their neck back or their collar brushes against that straight edge-line, to some extent, it always goes back to its ducktail way of laying. Those with this kind of neck hair have had years to adjust to a neckline that has a "mind of its own", so there won't be a major disappointment when you prove you're not a magician.

Up to this point, the edging has been done in a fairly consistent sequence of cuts around the head. If you were to go ahead with the left side of the neck's edging now, you would find it difficult to finish this edging at the right place on the back edge of the ear. So we jump ahead a little.

7..Left Sideburn. If you trimmed the right sideburn, you have a little snipping to do on the left. Do it the same way as the right side, except that here, if the scissor-and-comb method is used, do the upside-down comb handling on the front side of the burns.

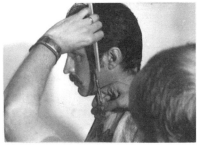

Whatever methods are used, trim it on both sides.

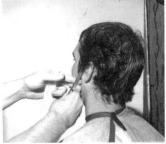 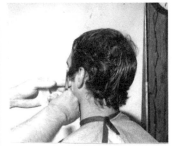

8. Left Side Hair. Before you start, comb the hair above the ear in a forward and down direction, as you did it on the right side. Then go back to the right side and comb that hair down into a pull-and-cut holding position so you can see exactly where the edge line was cut there in relation to the ear. Return to the left and repeat the same edging line on this side.

Do this cutting the same way it was done on the right side, but here, the first pull-and-cut is done to the hair that comes down over the ear. Work from there, cut by cut, toward the face.

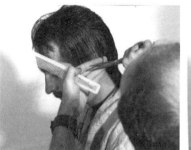 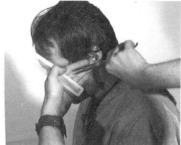

9. Left side neck. This part of the edge-cutting can now be done with greater assurance the edge-line starts off and ends up where you want it.

On the first pull-and-cut, use the cut hair that covers the ear as guide-hair (on this side, the guide-hair is at the "V" of the holding fingers). Remember to do the pull-and-cut on the inside of the holding fingers.

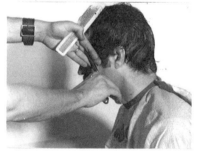 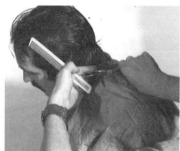

Be sure to keep in mind and duplicate the edge-line you cut on the right side of the neck. After the bottom is reached, round off the corner as you did on the right side.

10. Left side temple hair. For this last part of the edging, stand in a 10 - 11 o'clock position. Do the cutting the same way it was on the right side--the difference here is your cutting goes from the bottom toward the top

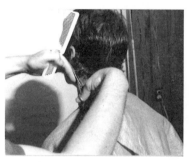 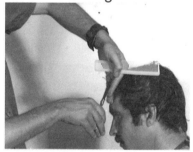

Lower temple.   Upper temple if needed.

The last of the edging is the corner where the lower temple and side hair meet. On this side I use the finger-bracing method after the side hair has been combed toward the corner. You can also use the pull-and-cut or the scissors-and-comb method.

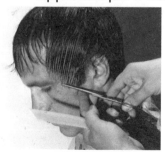

The edging.is done. Give yourself a few pats on the back, then it"s on to the last step.

***

Life is too short to smoke.   Bumper sticker

7.8 FINISHING TOUCHES

The finishing touches are to a haircut like gift wrapping is to a nice gift. We begin with last minute hair concerns for the fellows.
• **Extraneous hairs**.Post-adolescent males may need extra hair growth trimmed at the eyebrows, ears, and nose (see chapter 5 for the how-to).
• **Neck hair**. Extra hairs at the bottom and sides of neck can be cut shorter in several ways (page 78 described a couple of methods). Here I use close-cutting clippers to remove those extra hairs. The clipper is positioned as shown, then it moves downward.

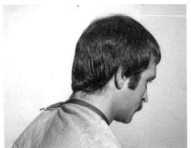
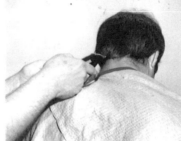
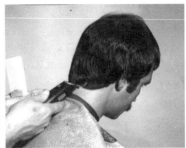

The before   The cutting

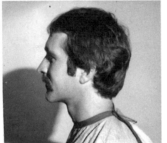
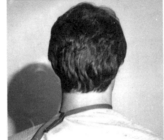

The same results are achieved by using soap lather and a razor. Start shaving where the scissor cutting left off.

The finished product

A growing number of fellows prefer the same scissors-over-comb cutting that women usually have done to their extra neck hairs. This approach, like eyebrow trimming, leaves the hair fairly short, but not with a freshly cut appearance. A little scissor over comb cutting leaves those neck hairs short, but not cut to the skin.
• **Trimming the beard**. When you give a haircut to a gent with a beard, you usually find that the beard no longer fits the new haircut. It is time to do some more trimming--the last chapter goes into detail.
Now we do those finishing touches that apply to all your haircuts.
1. Check for Longer Hairs in Front of the Ears. Repeat the combing technique shown for the right side hair (page 112) to be sure no longer hairs appear around the ear area.
2. **Back of the Ear Surplus**. Try as I may, I often end up with a chunk of longer hairs where the covering-the-ear edge line meets the side-of-the-neck edge line. To take care of that, I use what I call the "pinch-pull-cut" method.

***

You can always tell a real friend: when you make a fool of yourself, he doesn't feel you've done a permanent job.
Laurence J. Peter

When you're with someone and silence is comfortable, you are with a friend. Anonymous

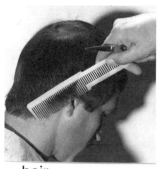 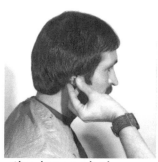 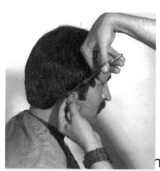

This method can be used anywhere around the edges where longer hairs show up.

hair   the longer hairs   and thumb as possible

3. Tapering the Hair that Covers the Ear. If you cut off 3/4 inch or more during the edging on the hair that covers the ear, that hair will be in the same condition neck hair is in after doing the first step in the 2-step tapering method. To remove this flippy prone hair, use the same diagonal cutting approach used during the second part of the tapering. Just a little tapering done to the longer hairs from above leaves the hair lying smoothly.

4. The Final Eyeballing. After you have dried the hair, comb or brush the hair into its preferred lying position. Look in a backbar mirror or step back a couple of yards. Check for a sloping neckline, uneven bangs, or unevenness anywhere it may show itself. Also look for any heaviness or cutting lines that might be left from the bulk-removal. As page 77 pointed out, when making corrections on straighter hair, you comb out the hair above on the sides and back sections, and behind on the top section from where you see the unevenness. The general rule to follow with flippy hair is to cut it a little shorter-- the exception occurs with coarse, straight hair and a ducktail neckline, here you leave the hair extra long or it must be cut extra short.

5. The Fun Part. With the hair combed or brushed so those ends are like carefully positioned shingles, show your patron a hand mirror. (A hand mirror used with a wall mirror allows them to see the back of the head.) Take the time to show them what a healthful scalp massage is, followed by a hand combing. Show them the mirror again- the contrast between the hair before cutting, and what they see now, makes it obvious a precision haircut makes all the difference.

6. Healthy Haircare. Share what you know about hair damage and how easy it is to make hair as healthy as can be. Keep in mind that if hair has been damaged by chemicals, heat appliances, thinning shears or razor cutting, the hair probably needs I or 2 more haircuts before the damaged hair is grown out enough to be all cut off. During this time, the customer must change their damaging ways if they are to correct their condition. Healthy haircare is simple, but it needs to be practiced daily.

There you have it, the world's most commonly given haircut. I recommend you stay with it until you're thoroughly comfortable with the haircutting process. After you have worked off your rough edges on this versatile haircut, you'll be ready for the more difficult haircuts. You will advance, but you'll come back to this cut again and again--this basic cut will always be in demand.

CHAPTER 8 LONG, LAYERED HAIRCUT

8.1 INTRODUCTION

This chapter teaches the best (to my way of thinking) and most skilled way of giving a long haircut. First you'll learn the most common version of a long, layered cut, along with the new ways of using your hands and tools. Then I show some of the different ways this basic haircut can be shaped. Concentrate your beginner's efforts on the first haircut--with that experience in your bag of skills, the later variations can be handled. These first photos reveal the transformation this haircut creates. The last row of photos on the next page show only the finished product (while busy working at the haircut shop, sometimes the before photo doesn't come to mind until after the cutting is done).

Flat line shape with the top, center path cut to a 3 inch length.

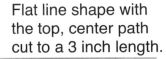
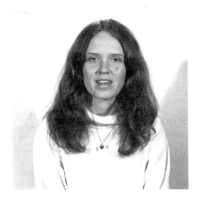
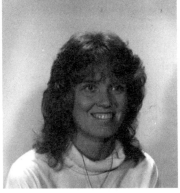
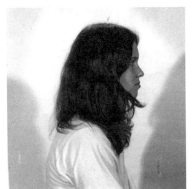
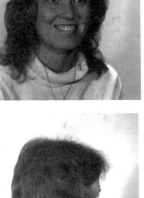
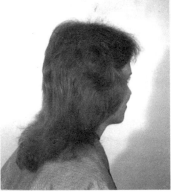
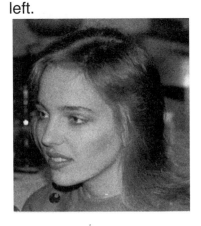

Type 2, straight, fine hair. Front hairline cowlick and ducktail. Same cut as one on left.

Cross between Type 1 and 2, slightly wavy, medium texture. Has only had perimeter trims in the past.

.

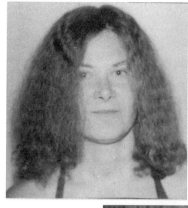
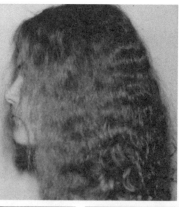
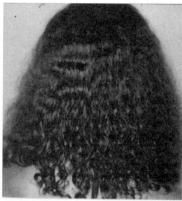

Type 2, extra wavy, medium hair.

Cut to 3 inch length on top, center path. Flat line shape.

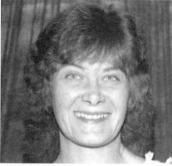
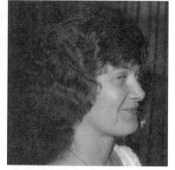
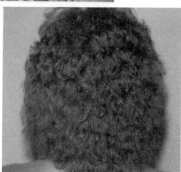

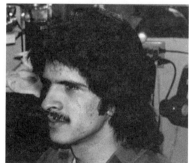
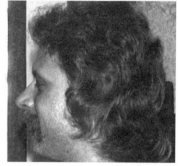
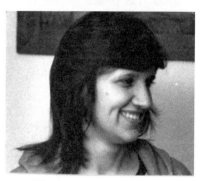

Type 2, straight, medium hair. 2 1/2 inches on top 3 paths Umbrella shape.

Type 1, wavy, medium hair. 2 inches on top, center path. Flat line shape.

Type 1, straight, medium to coarse hair. 3 1/2 inch top, center path, flat line shape.

The first chapter described how there are two basic ways to cut long hair. The easy way for the haircutter is the perimeter trim: the hair is combed down and snipped off on the bottom edges. A long, layered cut isn't as easy to cut, but it's much easier to care for on a daily basis. The easy haircut leaves a lot of hair on the head.

***

I expect to pass through life but once. If therefore, there be any kindness I can show, or any good thing I can do to any fellow being, let me do it now, and not defer or neglect it, as I shall not pass this way again.

William Penn

It is only with the heart that one can see rightly; what is essential is invisible to the eye.

Antoine de Saint Exupery

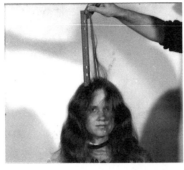

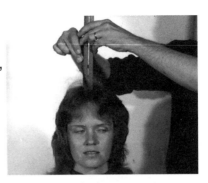

With the long, layered cut, over half of this top hair is cut off, but the way it's shaped and the precision cutting makes the hair look long.

While this haircut can't be braided or put into much of a ponytail as can the perimeter haircut, its lack of tangles and snarls and other easy care features makes it, like the equal-length cut, another people-pleaser.

8.2 SOME CHANGES FROM THE EQUAL-LENGTH HAIRCUT

With the equal-length cut, all the left hand had to do was lock into the same length-producing position while conforming to the shape of the head throughout the bulk-removal. With this long cut, your hand still operates as a spacer tool while holding the hair away from the head, but there are some differences.
• The bottom of the left hand won't always have the head to rest on.
• On some parts of the haircut, the hair is held out from the head in a different direction.
• The sequence of cuts is similar to the equal-length cut, but there are major changes.
•The edging conforms to the overall shape of the bulk-cutting, instead of to the hairline.

8.3 THE CUTTING LINE

The shortest hair is on top of the head--the farther down you go, the longer it gets:

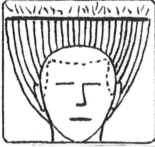
Cutting line

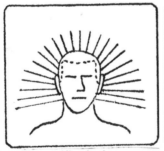
Electrified shape

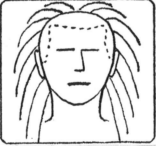
Lying naturally

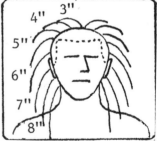
Typical lengths

This haircut would be extra easy if the customer could be hung upside-down during your cutting.

Just brush the hair down, and let gravity keep it that way as the hair is cut straight across-- as if you were cutting an upside down hedge.

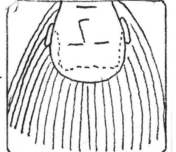

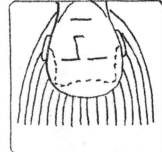

Without the convenience of this haircutting position, your haircutting efforts get a little difficult, but still very achievable. On the first long, layered cut, you'll go after the same flat cutting line shown on the upside-down model. However, you'll handle the hair in some new ways to make the cutting line happen with a person in the upright position.

8.4 CUT-BY-CUT BULK-REMOVAL

A. Preliminary Cutting

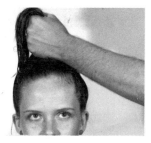
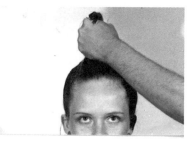

Removing hard-to-handle hair is easy with this technique. Just brush all of the hair up to the top center of the head as if there was to be a pony-tail up there. Then cut all the hair above the hand. This one-snip approximate cutting leaves the hair much easier to handle. Do this whenever you have 2 or more inches of hair to cut off. Leave the hair at least two inches longer than what is wanted for the final length. Preliminary edging makes long haircuts easier, but it's not necessary when you give the one-snip cut.

B. Cutting the Top

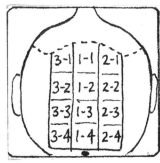

These are the same first 3 paths, with the same sequence of cuts in the paths, that were used on the equal-length cut.

Pathway 1 Hold the left hand straight up (perpendicular) from the scalp and rest the hand on the scalp. This leaves the hair about 3 inches long--a length that usually works well. Section 6-A shows a shorter cutting on top

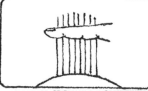
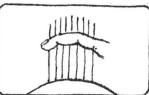

Due to the flat cutting line, your holding fingers are held straight across rather than conforming to the shape of the head (as they did on the equal-length cut). Stand at a 6 o'clock position and comb the top hair forward. The first photo shows how to make the hair easier to handle for the first comb up and cut.

***

The person who says it cannot be done should not interrupt the person doing it.

Chinese proverb

He is well paid that is well satisfied.

William Shakespeare

If you want to leave your footsteps in the sands of time, wear work shoes. Anonymous

Without work all life goes rotten.

Albert Camus

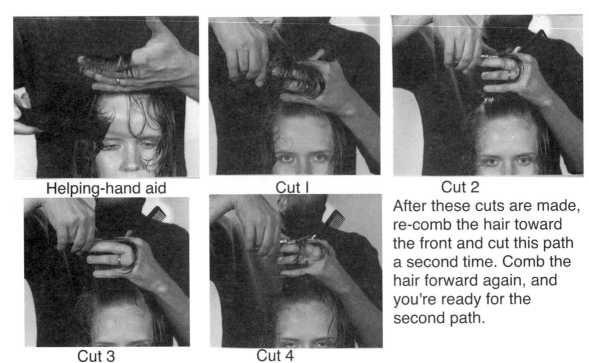

Helping-hand aid Cut I Cut 2

After these cuts are made, re-comb the hair toward the front and cut this path a second time. Comb the hair forward again, and you're ready for the second path.

Cut 3 Cut 4

Pathwav 2 Depending on how flat or oval the top of the head is, you may only have the wrist resting on the head while cutting this path. In any case, continue the flat cutting line established on the first pathway's cutting. To that end you have two important aids:
(I) Be sure the comb up includes some of the first pathway 's already-cut hair. That helpful guide-hair in your holding hand's grasp shows you how much to cut off.
(2) Keep a clear mental picture of the flat cutting line you want, with your holding fingers held just below that line.

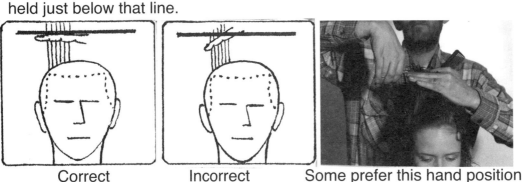

Correct Incorrect Some prefer this hand position

For myself, the more relaxed position shown in the cut-by-cut photos works best.

***

Information's pretty thin stuff unless mixed with experience. Clarence Day

Honor lies in honest toil. Grover Cleveland

Life is a succession of lessons, which must be lived to be understood. Ralph Waldo Emerson

You have reached the pinnacle of success as soon as you become uninterested in money, compliments, or publicity. Dr. O. A. Battista

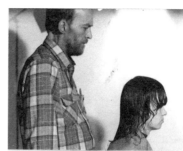

To help you keep this cutting line in mind, do the top cutting with the chair in a high position. A lower position may be less arm-tiring, but when you look down on the top, it's much easier to get away from the flat cutting line we are after.

As this first photo shows, you can stand at a 1 o'clock position and use the comb away method. My preference shows after the first cut.

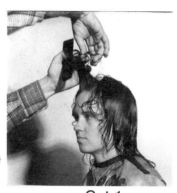

Cut 1

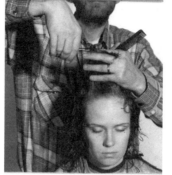

Cut 2

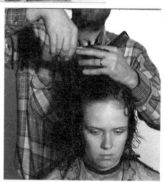

Cut 3

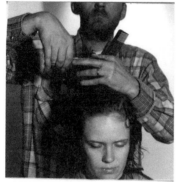

Cut 4

The arrow points to guide-hair at the "V" of the holding fingers when standing at 6 o'clock. If you're at 1 o'clock using the comb-away method, the guide-hair is at the finger tips.

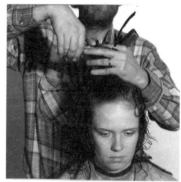

Guide hair at the "V"

Pathway 3 This last top pathway, like the second, can be done from either a front or back position. I prefer 11 o'clock and use the comb-away method.

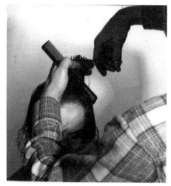

Cut I

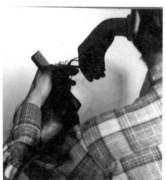

Cut 2

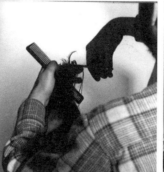

Cut 3

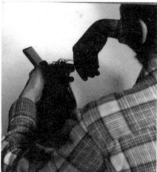

Cut 4

Before moving on to the next part, go back and repeat each of the cuts in pathways 2 and 3. The idea is to be sure this first part of the haircut is done as well as possible because that top hair is much used as guide-hair for the cutting you do next.

If the hair were electrified after the top three pathways have been cut, it would appear something like this:

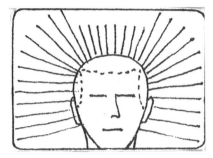

The next part of the haircut removes this unevenness. At the same time, the hair around the sides and back will be evenly-cut with a gradually increasing length to it.

C. Sides and Back

The equal-length haircut had a next-door-neighbor sequence of paths around the sides and back of the head. Each pathway had 2 to 6 cuts as you moved through the paths. With the long, layered cut you follow the same sequence of pathways, but instead of 2 - 6 cuts, you comb up all of the hair in the pathway--up to the already-cut top hair--and cut it off with just one snip.

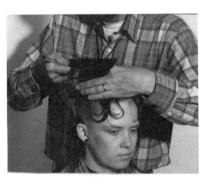

For your best vision and tool handling ease, have your customer in a low sitting position and stand at 9 o'clock. With some head bending help, the line of vision shown here works best.

This is how you go about it:

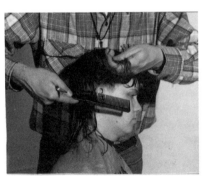
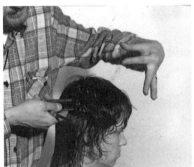
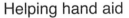

Helping hand aid   Combing up   Grasp the hair
                              ***

To learn and from time to time apply what one has learned--isn't that a pleasure?
Confucius
Ralph Waldo Emerson

Skill to do comes of doing.

He is well paid that is well satisfied.
William Shakespeare

Change how you see not how you look.
Bumper sticker

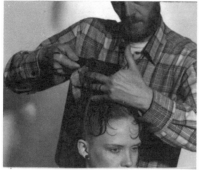
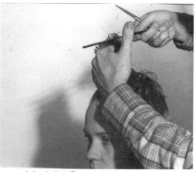
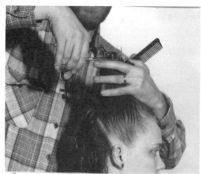

| Slide your left hand up to cutting position | Hold. Comb goes to the resting place | The cut |

1. How Much to Cut Off? To cut off the right amount of side and back hair, comb up into the cut hair on the outside edge of the top section--this gets some of the already-cut top hair (guide-hair) in your grasp. That guide-hair is easily seen if you stand on the side opposite that part of the head you're working on. For example, if you're cutting the right side hair, stand to the person's left; when you work on the back, you stand in front.

With the equal-length cut, the guide-hair always appeared at the 'V" or out at the finger tips.

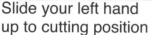

Now it shows up as short hairs against a background of longer hairs.

It takes careful combing to get the guide-hair into your grasp, and you need to look closely to see it. Cut off all the longer hairs that protrude above the shorter guide-hair. Take care not to cut any of those helpful hairs.

2. Positioning your left hand. Once you have the long side hair and the short top hair in your hand, slide your spacer tool (with a pinching pressure between the holding fingers) straight up until you have 1/8 - 1/4 inch of guide-hair protruding above the holding fingers.

At this point your holding fingers are just beneath the flat cutting line. Use this first more relaxed position, or the flat hand approach shown in the second photo.

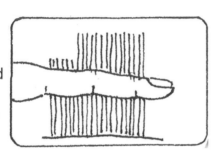
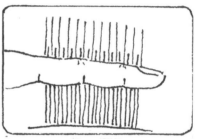

3. Comb Handling. You will deal with some long, cumbersome hair when you comb up the pathways around the sides and back. The preliminary cutting minimizes this, and to make it easier when you begin the comb up, make good use of the helping-hand aid and the sideways method of starting out above the ear. There are a few more things to know about the comb handling you'll do.

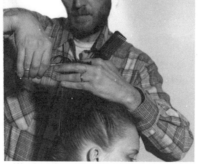

Uncovering the guide-hair. After the sides or back hair is combed up, and the holding hand slides up to the cutting position, the longer uncut hair may "flop" over and cover the guide-hair when the comb is transferred to its resting place. The remedy is easy: comb the long hairs away from you and the covered-up guide-hair is exposed. Now the comb goes to its resting place and the cutting can proceed.

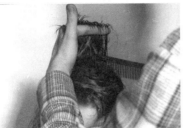

The guide-hair is covered up

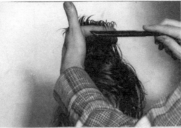

Flip your wrist so the teeth of the comb are pointed away

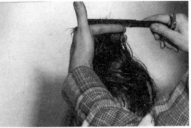

Comb through the hair so the guide-hair is exposed

The hairs that don't reach up to the cutting. You may find some of the lower hair (the hair toward the bottom of the path you comb up) is not long enough to reach up to the top area for cutting. Don't worry about those hairs. All you have to be concerned with is the hair that's long enough to reach the flat cutting line. With this way of shaping the hair, those shorter hairs blend in very well.

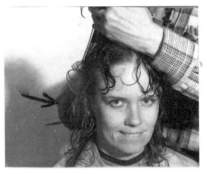

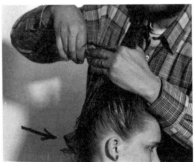

Too much hair. When you gave the equal-length cut, you were cautioned about trying to get too much hair into your grasp. The length and amount of hair being combed up around the sides and back on this haircut is such that you can't be concerned about this "overloading" problem-the unevenness that results from this is smoothed off later.

The head gets moved.
You always have to move the person's head around during any haircut to achieve easy comb-handling and maximum vision. This haircut requires more than the usual head-bending cooperation as you comb up the hair around the sides and back.

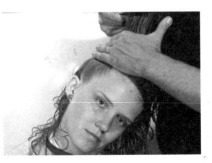

A different combing. On the equal-length cut, the sides and back hair is combed down before beginning a pathway up through the hair. On this cut, the more the hair can stay combed up after a comb up and cut, the easier it is.

***

The real art of conversation is not only to say the right thing at the right time, but to leave unsaid the wrong thing at the tempting moment.

Sign in a diner

4. The Sequence of Pathways Around the Head

This is the way you'll work around the head. One long comb up and cut takes care of each path.

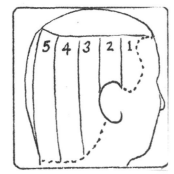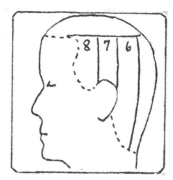

Pathway 1 The first comb up and cut off is done to the same front right-side pathway used on the equal-length haircut's right section.

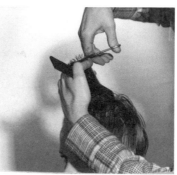

After this first cut is made, the rest of the pathways you comb up and cut will have an extra guide-hair aid to rely on. In addition to combing up the hair so some cut hair from the top section is included, also **overlap** the comb up so you're including a little of the path that was just cut.

As you see, on the second pathway's comb up and cut, the extra guide-hair comes from where your second path overlaps the first path. You will be able to employ this extra help on the second path, and on all remaining pathways around the head.

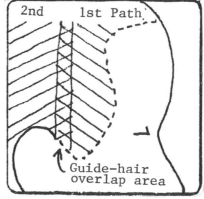

When you carefully comb up the hair on the second pathway, the hair between your holding fingers will include:
(1) guide-hair from the overlap area,
(2) guide-hair from the already-cut top section, and
(3) hairs to be cut.

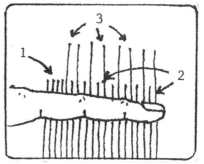

***

Whatever I do, I give up my whole self to it.　　　　　　Edna St.Vincent Millay

This photo and the blow-up clearly show the double guide hair. The arrows point to the guide hair from the side's first pathway and the guide hair from the top section.

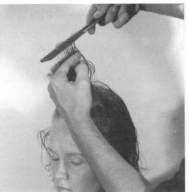
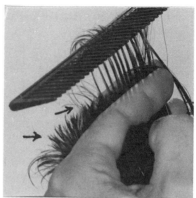

The reason for overlapping the paths is that it insures all the hair long enough to reach to the top is cut--you can't miss a hair.

Pathways 2 - 8 The first pathway's comb up and cut was shown on the previous page. Here we continue the trip around the head.

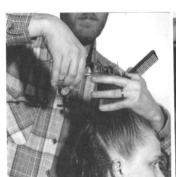
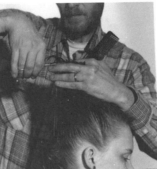
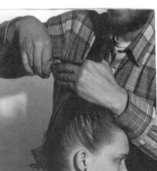
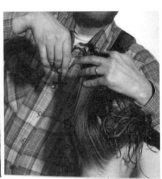

| Path 2 | Path 3 | Path 4 | Path 5 |

Step over to the customer's right and finish your cuts.

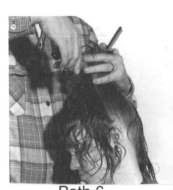
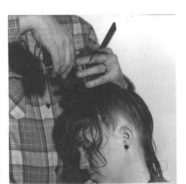
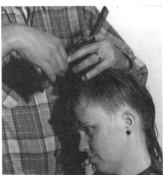

| Path 6 | Path 7 | Path 8 |

The exact number of paths depends on head and holding hand size.

Now go back to path I, and do your second-time-through cutting by repeating all of the cuts around the head. **Only** cut off the stragglers.

***

Through perseverance many people win success out of what seemed to be certain failure.
Benjamin Disraeli

Trust your hunches. They're usually based on facts filed away just below the conscious level.
Joyce Brothers

D. Smoothing Off

When you are finished with the top and sides/back parts of the bulk-removal, you'll find a little unevenness where these two parts of your cutting meet.

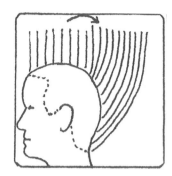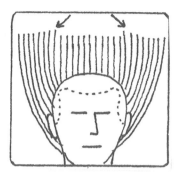

To deal with this unevenness, go through the same pathways 4 and 5 used on the equal-length haircut's top section. Here the comb is handled in a different way than was used on the equal-length cut: once the comb is positioned flat to the scalp (teeth lightly scraping the scalp), lift the comb in a **pivoting** manner like this on the fourth path.

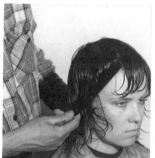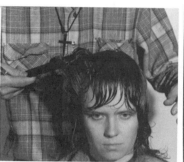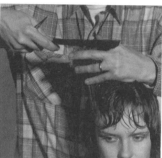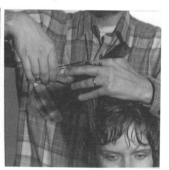

Do this smooth-off cutting with the chair in a high position.

Use the comb-away method for the cuts on the left side of the head. Keep in mind your flat cutting line, and place the top of your holding fingers just below that line.

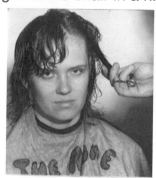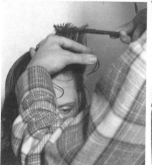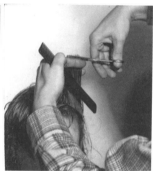

This smooth off cutting has a more familiar double guide-hair aid to use. The hair to be cut appears like this:

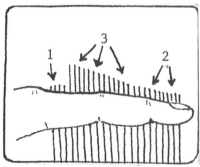

1. At the "V" of the fingers you'll have the already-cut, top section hair to use as a guide.
2. Out at the finger tips are the hair ends from the sides that are used as a second guide.
3. The hair between the two guides will be cut off.

***

Thinking is the talking of the soul with itself.

Plato

Pathway 4. The first cut is shown on the previous page. The rest of the cuts go like this:

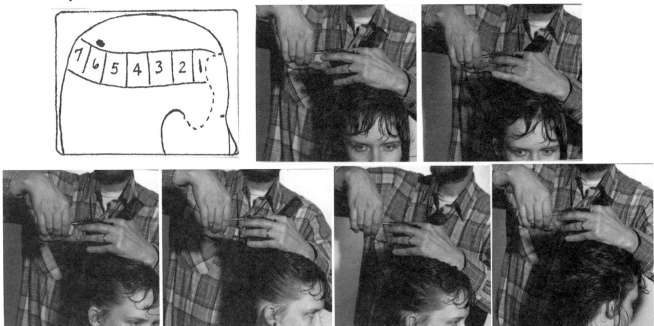

Finish pathway 5 using the comb-away (the first cut is shown on the previous page).

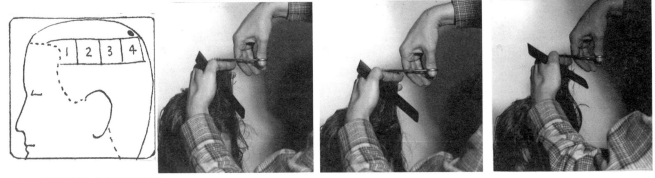

8.5 EDGE-CUTTING

The edge-cutting for the long, layered cut differs significantly from the way it was done on the equal-length cut.

A. Methods to Use

While the equal-length and short, full cuts need a variety of edge cutting techniques to trim those perimeter hairs evenly, with the long, layered cut just the pull-and-cut method. can be used. (Force of habit usually has me using the modified-bulk-removal technique on the bangs and temple region hair, but it's not necessary.)

***

Before I judge my neighbor, let me walk a mile in his moccasins.   Sioux proverb

If you judge people you have no time to love them.   Mother Teresa

Unless each day can be looked back upon by an individual as one in which he has had some fun, some joy, some real satisfaction, that day is a loss.   Dwight Eisenhowe

B. Shape of the Cutting Line

When you did the edging on the equal-length cut, the hair was combed straight out from the hairline and cut so the edge line was, by and large, equal distance from the hairline. With our long cut you also comb the hair fairly straight out and away from the hairline to make the cuts, but because of the increasing length of the hair, you cut the edge line so it conforms to this increasing length on the sides.

To get this cutting to go along with the bulk-cutting, you must do the edging around the face in the shape of a Christmas tree.

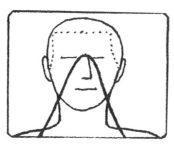

This tree shape is achieved, snip-by-snip, while the top and side hair is combed forward and held toward the lower part of the face.

C. The Cutting Position Versus the Lying Position

Back in chapter 5, I explained how the final lying position for the edge hair would shrink up and be shorter than the hair is while being cut. This rule of haircutting is even more noticeable when you do the edging on the long, layered cut, especially if the hair has a Type 2 grain or if it's wavy or curly. Straighter types of hair with a Type 1 hair grain are not affected by this shrinking edge line as much; but, to be on the safe side, you should make your edge cuts at least 2 inches longer than the lying position you want for the edge hair. Curlier hair or hair with a Type 2 grain needs as much as 4 inches of extra length. You can always cut off more later, but once it is gone,...

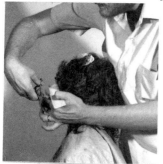
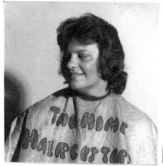
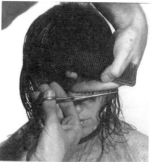
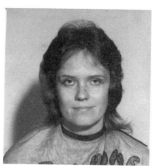

Cutting versus lying position   Cutting versus lying position

The difference between the position of the cutting line and the final lying position is especially noticeable on the hair that frames the face--that hair normally lies toward the back of the head, but the cutting is done with the hair pulled forward.

D. How It's Done

Cutting the long, layered cut's edge line just requires an awareness of the Christmas tree shape to be strived for. Cut with this shape in mind while the hair is pulled forward in the general direction of the lower half of the center of the face.

1. Sequence of Cuts. The preliminary or final edging for the long, layered cut always starts at the top of the tree and continues down the person's right side to the longest hair at the back of the head. Then back to the treetop and down and around the left side. Remember, when you do the bulk-cutting for this haircut (as with the other layered cuts), the edge hairs are already cut and in the basic shape you want. When doing the final edging you only cut off a little unevenness. This sequence of cuts allows you to comb a little of the already-cut edge hair into your hand's grasp on each cut made after the first one. Be sure to use that guide-hair.

Starting at the top of the "tree" stand at a 12 or 1 o'clock position for the pull-and-cut, or a 3 or 4 o'clock spot for the modified-bulk-removal. Assuming your top center path was cut to the 3 inch length and you're working with an average hairline in front, the hair at the treetop will lie at the bridge of the nose. Comb the hair from the crown region to the front where the left hand waits to grasp the hair--use this lengthy combing for each cut.

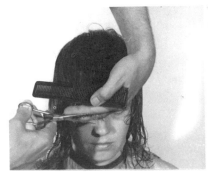 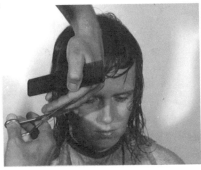 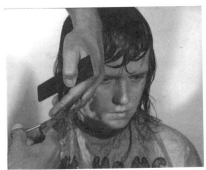

| Cut 1 | Cut 2 | Cut 3 |

After you cut the upper part of the tree on the right side, use the pull-and-cut on the rest of the cuts you make on the trip to the middle of the back hair. The following photos show the cutting done above the holding fingers: remember to make your cuts with the preferred, safer way with the cuts made on the inside of the fingers.

***

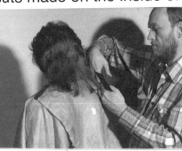

These cuts need to have a straight-on line of vision. The chair should be in a high position or both could stand.

Man--despite his artistic pretensions, his sophistication, and his accomplishments--owes his existence to a six-inch layer of top soil and the fact it rains.

Anonymous

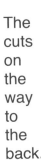

The cuts on the way to the back.

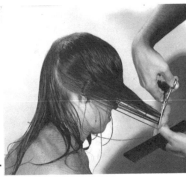 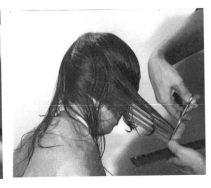 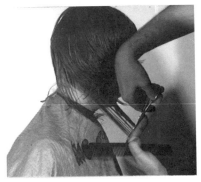

***

To own a bit of ground, to scratch it with a hoe, to plant seeds, and watch the renewal of life--this is the commonest delight of the race, the most satisfying thing a man can do.

Charles Dudley Warner

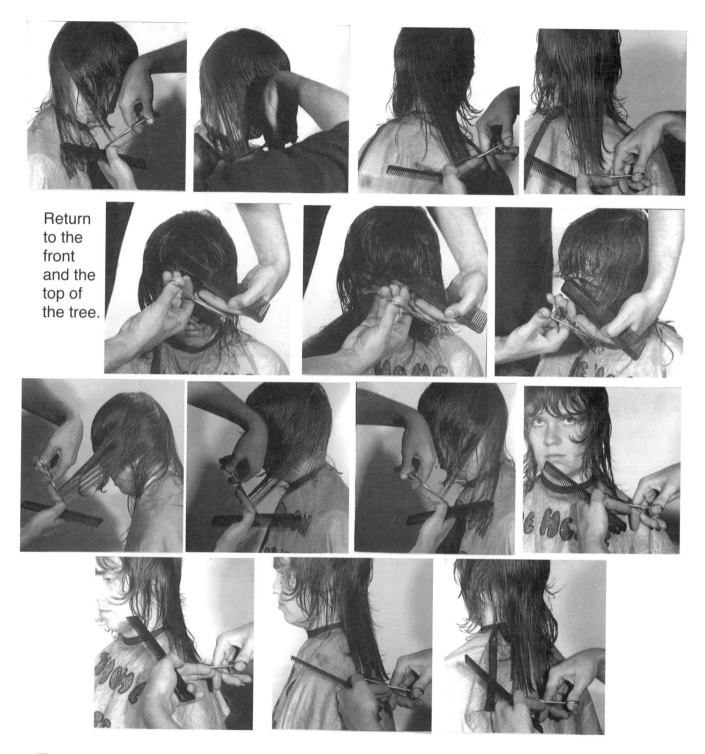

Return to the front and the top of the tree.

To match the edge-cutting line on the left side to the right side, do the following:
• Remember, cut off a minimum of hair and use that guide-hair.
• Keep a mental picture of where your left (hair holding) hand was positioned on the right side in relation to the features of the face (nose, mouth, chin, neck and shoulder) and duplicate those positions on the left side.
• If one side is a little shorter than the other when the hair is in its normal lying state, trim the longer side to match the shorter. Page 140 has more on checking the length.

2. Side Part. Flat shaping and Christmas tree edging works well if the hair has a center or somewhat off-center part. If the hair grain dictates a side part, the umbrella version of a long, layered cut or the combination cut (see sections 6-B and C in this chapter) are well-suited, but they are the shortest of the long cuts--maybe too short for your client. If you give the flat shaped version to hair with a side part, the Christmas tree edging is done as previously shown, then make some modifications:
• Find the natural part and comb the top toward its preferred lying side.

• Trim that portion of the bangs closest to the part so those hairs are as short as the top of the tree hairs.

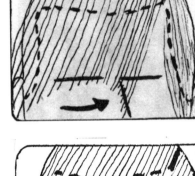 -->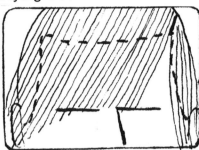

• Then trim the upper temple region hairs a little so they blend with the shorter bangs. Trimming the first few inches of the upper side hair removes the unevenness.

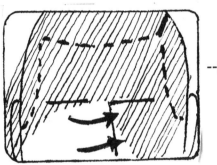 -->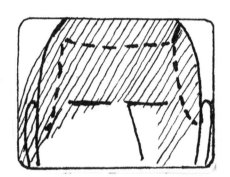

8.6 MODIFYING THE LONG, LAYERED CUT

These ways to modify a long, layered cut are arranged from the easiest to the more difficult. While the first option can be used with your initial haircuts, I don't recommend the others until you're comfortable with the haircut shown in the cut-by-cut photos.

A. A Shorter Overall Length
The length the hair is left on the top pathways determines the overall length of a long, layered haircut. This is due to the way the sides and back are pulled up and cut while using the top hair as a guide for how much is cut off. A shorter cutting on top leaves all the hair shorter; a longer cutting on top leaves all the hair longer.
A shorter cutting on top doesn't require any changes from how the bulk-removal was done on the longer cut shown earlier. A flat cutting is still the goal, the only difference is a shorter length-producing position for your left hand while cutting the top. This shorter cutting keeps the bottom of your hand resting on the scalp while cutting the top section's second and third paths. The shorter top also keeps the hand resting on the scalp as the sides and back hair are pulled up for cutting.

***

Next time you feel like complaining, remember your garbage can eats better than 30% of the world's population.

Anonymous

Because of the shorter length, your edge-cutting line is altered to some extent. The Christmas tree edge line needs to be higher on the forehead, and wider at the top.

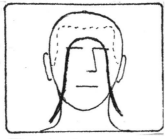

The short approach

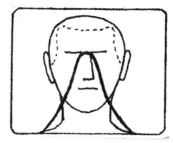

A longer cutting

This shorter cutting is well-suited to fine hair, or the wavier, curly, and kinky types of hair. The finer or curlier the hair, the shorter it can be cut: you can go as short as 1 inch on the first path, but 1 1/2 to 2 inches usually works best. (If the top hair is cut extra short and you want to leave the bangs longer, refer to page 105 for the how-to.) Keep in mind that straight, coarse textured hair may not lie well if cut much shorter than 3 inches.

B. Umbrella Shape

This way to shape hair, when combined with a shorter cutting on top, produces the shortest version of the long, layered cut.

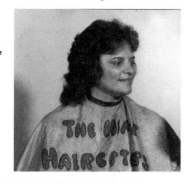

***

Plant your own garden and decorate your own soul, instead of waiting for someone to bring you flowers.

Anonymous

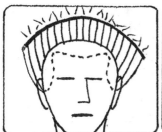
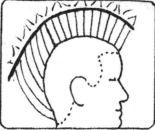
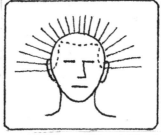
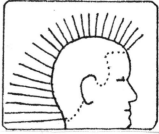

Cutting line   Electrified shape

1. Bulk-Removal for the Umbrella Cutting

This haircut's top 3 paths are done the same way as the equal-length cut's first 3 paths: the holding fingers conform to the head's shape. With every head somewhat rounded on top, when you begin with an equal length cutting on the top 3 pathways, you create a rounded cutting line. The cutting line on the sides and back is a fairly straight line that slopes downward--it continues the cutting line established on the top 3 pathways. Because of this, the shape of the top of the head does affect the overall cutting line.

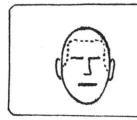
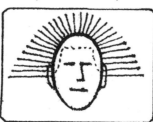
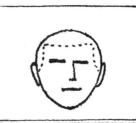
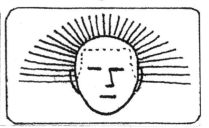

Part 1 Cut the top three paths with the holding fingers conforming to the shape of the head. After these paths are cut, the electrified shape shows what's next. The next part removes this unevenness and shapes the rest of the hair.

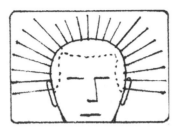

Part 2 Follow the same pathways and long comb up used on the first long cut's sides and back hair. Due to the equal-length cutting on the top three paths, you'll be able to rest the bottom of your hand on the scalp, instead of holding it out in space.

Now the bottom of the left hand can rest on the head.

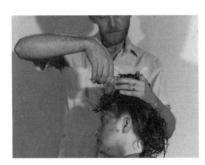

With flat line shaping, the hand is floating, and only the wrist or forearm rests on the head.

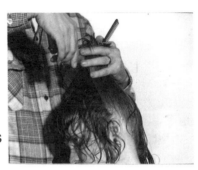

Part 3 Use the "pivoting" comb manipulation as you follow the same sequence of cuts used on the fourth and fifth paths for the equal-length haircut. After these cuts are made, additional pathways 6 and 7 (just below and parallel to 4 and 5) may also be necessary. All of the cutting in this part of the haircut has your holding fingers sloped downward instead of being held straight out as they were for the flat shaping on the first long-layered cut. Rest the bottom of your left hand or wrist on the top side of the head.

With this cutting, like the smooth off cuts on the first long-layered cut, remove only a little unevenness that results from the part 1 and part 2 cutting.

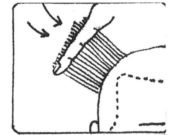

2. Edging
The edging shape for this cut reflects the shorter bulk-removal on the sides of the top section. Here your Christmas tree gets a "fatter" edge-cutting line.

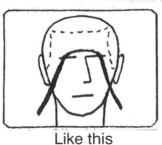
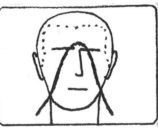

Like this   Not like this

This version of the long cut works well with any hair, but it's extra well-suited to wavy or curlier hair, and fine hair with a Type 2 hair grain.

C. Combination Cut

This long haircut's bulk-removal is a mixture of an equal-length cut and a long, layered cut; if you choose an edging treatment to the hair around the ears like that shown in the example, your combination cut borrows something from all three layered haircuts. This way to shape the hair has the extra easy-care features of the shorter equal-length haircut, and a somewhat longer look of a long, layered cut.

The combination cut is similar to the equal-length cut that has the back hair shaped longer. But there are some new "twists" to this cutting, and the overall appearance is considerably longer:

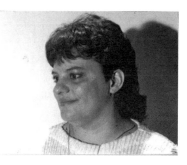 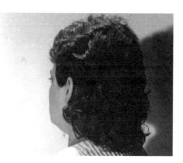

1. Bulk-Removal

The bulk-cutting consists of two main parts and a third smooth off cutting.

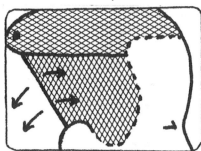

Part 1 First give an equal-length cutting (2 or 3 inches) to the top section, and to this portion of the side section:

For the side cutting, you need to part the hair from the rear upper ear to the crown.

Part 2 The bulk-removal on the back can be done several ways--the longer cutting approaches are extra adaptable to straighter hair, the shorter approaches work on any type of hair, but especially curlier hair. These options are arranged from longest to shortest:

• Pathway by pathway, pull up and cut off the back section hair as you did for the flat shaping of the long, layered cut.

• Make a path around the upper 2 - 3 inches of the back so it has a gradually increasing length-the same way it's done for the umbrella version. Then pull up the back hair (pathway by pathway) to the bottom of this path and cut off the excess back length.

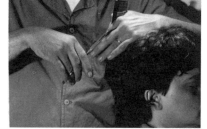

• Repeat the second option, but make one more path just below and parallel to the path around the upper back. Pull up the lower back hair and cut it while using the bottom of this second path as a guide for how much is cut off.

Part 3 The area where you go from an equal-length cutting on the sides to the increasing length around the upper back needs more than the usual smoothing off cuts

***

Three things in human life are important: the first is to be kind, the second is to be kind, and the third is to be kind.

Henry James

to make it blend together. This area needs the holding fingers positioned so they go along with the increased length on the back hair, while you also have some of the shorter side hair in your grasp.

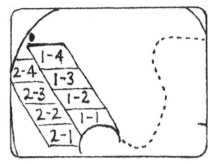

This cutting can be done with a horizontal positioning of your left hand while standing at the opposite side of the head. However, it may be easier to employ the cutting technique used for approximate bulk-cutting (see page 56). This method has you stand on the same side you're working on. One path should do it, but two may be needed if the back hair was given one of the longer length producing options.

2. Edging

Cut the bangs and temple area as you did for the equal-length cut. The edging on the hair around the ears can be done so some part of the ear is left covered, or it can be cut so all of the ear shows (most prefer this second option).

Whichever option is chosen, don't cut any of the longer hair at the upper, back part of the ear. To explain how you go about it, both types of hair grain have to be looked at.

• **Type 2 hair grain**. Assume the bulk-cutting left the side hair 2 1/2 inches.

If you want to leave some of the ear covered, you can give it a straight-across edging line as used on the equal-length cut.

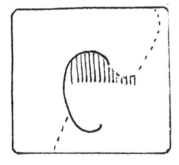

Or the edging line can follow the hairline above, and in front of the ear.

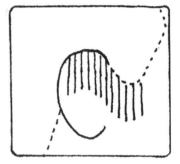

If all the ear is to be exposed, comb the side hair down, over the ear and cut off 1 - 1 1/2 inches of length so the edge line conforms to the hairline above and in front of the ear.

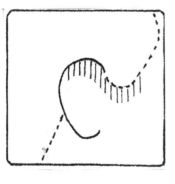

Comb side hair back--it rises up and sits on top of the ear. The hair at the dip (in front of the ear) can be cut as shown here, or it can be left as is.

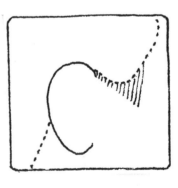

• **Type 1 hair grain**. With the hair growing straight down, you need to leave the hair longer to have it bend toward the back (the way most people like to wear this haircut). Again, we'll assume 2 1/2 inches of length from the bulk-cutting (3 inches maybe needed on coarser hair). If the side hair is to lie toward the back, give the edge hairs a minimum cutting with the edge line conforming to the hairline, from the dip to the top back of the ear. If the side hair is to lie downward, the edge line can be cut as short as you want--most prefer the straight-across cutting line. With either hair grain type, if 1 or

2 inches of the bottom side hair is cut off, that bottom hair needs to be tapered a little. (See the 2-step tapering method in the previous chapter.)

The edging that starts at the top, back of the ear and goes down the side of the neck is done much the same as you did it for an equal-length haircut with longer neck hair--the extra length of the back hair means your edge line is more toward the face. This edging needs to be a minimum cutting that reflects the increasing length of the back hair. Don't attempt to blend the shorter hair from above the ear with the longer hair from the back-- just pull that longer back hair forward and ignore the shorter hair. Do the edging on the back, bottom hair using the pull-and-cut. Most prefer this hair to be quite long, but it can be cut shorter than the minimum cutoff used on the side of the neck. After cutting across the bottom, round off the corners where the bottom meets the sides.

The combination cut is adaptable to any hair, but it's extra good for wavy or curly types of hair, or finer-textured straight hair with a Type 2 grain--the kind that flips forward in the lower temple area if left too long (page 169 has more on this condition).

D. An Extra Long Version

As explained earlier, the overall length of a long, layered cut depends on the length of the top hair. This longest of the layered haircuts is saved for last because the extra length on top means the left hand won't have anything to rest on during the bulk cutting--the hand holding the hair floats in space and arms get extra tired. The bulk-removal for this version is cut the same as for the basic long, layered haircut. The edge cutting-line is altered to conform to the longer bulk-cutting.

The Christmas tree's top is lower and the overall shape is skinnier than for the shorter versions.

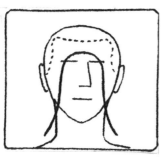 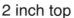 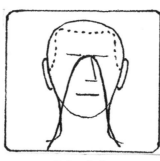 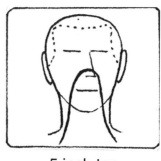

| 2 inch top | 3 inch top | 5 inch top |

The first of the three pathways on top can be left as long as 6 - 7 inches, but as this photo shows, 5 inches on the beginning path leaves plenty of extra length.

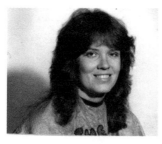

This longer cutting can be used with any hair; however, wavy hair or coarse, straight hair works best.

While this is the most challenging of the long haircuts, when you're comfortable with the earlier versions, you should be able to handle it.

***

Have patience with all things, but first of all with yourself.   St. Francis de Sales

8.7 CHECK FOR LENGTH EVENNESS

You easily checked the equal-length cut for consistent length by randomly pulling the hair straight out from the head in 10 to 12 places and measuring that hair with a ruler (or a comb that has measurement on the backbar). With the increasing lengths of long, layered cuts, you have to be exacting in where you do your checking. The parts of the head to be checked include the following:

• Sides. If you pick a checkpoint, say 2 inches above the ear, be sure to check the exact same spot on the other side.

• Top left checking requires a corresponding spot on the top right.

• Back section-left side versus the right side. Measure at points that are the same distance up from the hairline at both checkpoints

A little different way to check the hair length on the back is to grab a strand of 10 to 15 hairs behind both ears, at the same spot in relation to the ear. Pull those strands of hairs together so they meet at the spine--if they don't come together over the spine, that's telling you one side has been left longer than the other.

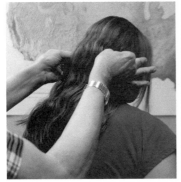
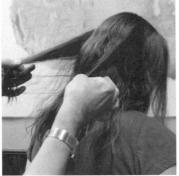
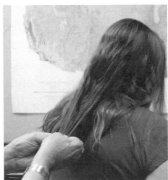

Pinch a strand of hairs behind each ear

Pull them together and downward

If it meets at the spine, it's cut right

If it meets to the left of the spine, the right side is longer than the left side-- a meeting to the right side says the left side has the longer hair.

(The length check shown above is also used on a long hair trim--see page 178.)

With the long, layered cut the tendency is to gradually leave the hair too long during the bulk-removal. For example, the first (right) side of the head is cut to the correct length, but when you get around to the left side, the hair is gradually longer. If you find an area longer than the other side of the head or section, go to the area that is shorter and check where your left hand is held when the hair is up in the cutting position: back to the longer area to recut with the correct position duplicated there.

When you have these long, layered ways of shaping hair in your bag of skills, you're ready for the last, most challenging of the three layered haircuts.

***

Inside every old person is a young person wondering what happened   Bumper sticker

Lord, help me to be the person my dog thinks I am   Bumper sticker

There is nothing like sealing a letter to inspire a fresh thought.   Anonymous

CHAPTER 9 SHORT, FULL HAIRCUT

9.1 INTRODUCTION

You need to know about short haircutting and some new ways to manipulate your hands. The cut-by-cut part of this chapter shows a somewhat longer (more full) version of a short haircut. It was chosen because it can be cut with just scissors and comb (no clippers needed), and because of its popularity. Later pages show variations of our main short haircut. As the photos show, this haircut can take on as many different looks.

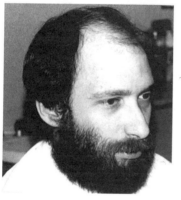

Top is cut to 1 3/4 inches; 3/4 inch around bottoms

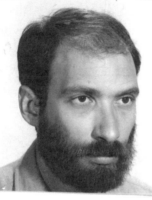

3 inch length on top; 1 inch around bottoms- shorter in front of ears. Bangs cut shorter than minimum cutting

Type 1, straight, medium texture. Thinning top needs shorter length

Type 2, extra wavy, medium texture

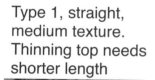

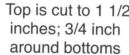

Top is cut to 1 1/2 inches; 3/4 inch around bottoms

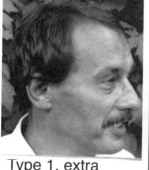

Cut to 1 3/4 inches on top; a little less than 3/4 inch at the bottoms

Type 1, extra fine, straight hair

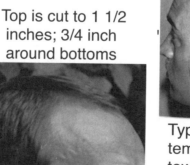

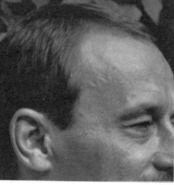

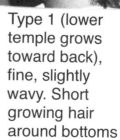

Type 1 (lower temple grows toward back), fine, slightly wavy. Short growing hair around bottoms

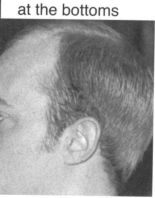

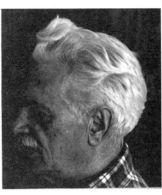

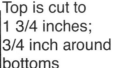

Top is cut to
1 3/4 inches;
3/4 inch around
bottoms

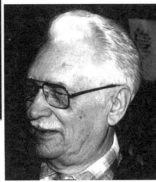

Type 2, slightly
wavy, medium
texture

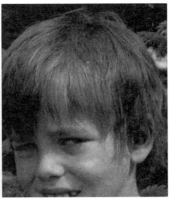

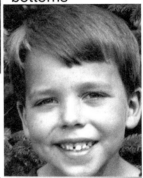

Top is 2 1/2
inches with
bangs trimmed
shorter than
minimum cutting;
3/4 inch around
bottoms

Type 1, straight,
medium texture.
Cowlick on front
hairline needs
extra top length

This shortest way to shape hair is taught last because it's the most difficult of the layered haircuts. There are two main reasons why this is such a challenging haircut:
•Because of the shortness of this cut, your cutting has to be extra precise. With a 2 or 3 inch equal-length cut, the hair can be left with unevenness (as much as a 1/4 inch, even 1/2 inch on curlier hair) and it won't show--you still have a well-done haircut. The long, layered cut has even more room for error. With the short, full haircut, any unevenness sticks out like a sore thumb. A cooperative customer who can hold their head still, and a very precise use of the hair holding hand is needed for success on this haircut.

• You'll be tapering a decreasing length to the hair around the sides and back. This tapering would be simple if a head of hair had the growing surface shown here. However, a typical head of hair has about 2 1/2 to 3 inches of growing surface on the sides and about 5 or 6 inches on the back.

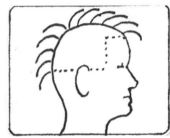

The top section gets a equal-length cutting, so the tapering begins with the same length (for example, 2 inches) all around the upper sides and back. From that length around the top, the hair is gradually cut shorter around the sides and back until the bottom hair is cut to a length of 3/4 inch or less. The difficulty comes from having to blend the tapering on the 3 inch long side sections and the 6 inch-long back section so it's all smoothly-cut. With the experience gained from the first two cuts and my how-to directions, you can expect excellent short cuts--the kind given by better professionals.

9.2 BULK-REMOVAL

A. Top Section
Short haircuts generally need the top hair cut on the shorter side (2 inches or less) to have the whole head of hair fit together--so the top is in balance with the shortness

around the lower portions of the hair. The top five pathways are cut like an equal-length haircut. (Page 152 shows how it's done if the top is left longer than 2 inches.)

B. Sides and Back

There are a number of ways to do the tapered cutting needed for this part of the haircut-the photos show my preferred method (see page 104 for other ways).

This haircut, perhaps more than the first two, needs you to clearly visualize the cutting line and shape wanted because the left hand gets into a variety of positions that produce a gradually decreasing length. The hair holding hand conforms to the shape of this cutting line as the hair is held straight out from the head. (See chapter 3 to review the cutting line for this haircut.)

Pathway 1 This path is just below and parallel to pathway 4 on the top section. The first few cuts in this right side pathway are slightly tapered. For example, the top is cut to a 2 inch length. Position your left hand so it leave the hair 2 inches long at the "V" of the holding fingers, and about 1 1/2 inch at the finger tips. Use the 2 inch long hair from the top section as guide-hair--it appears at the "V". The cutting goes like this:

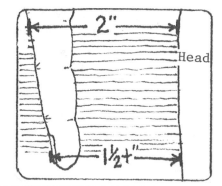

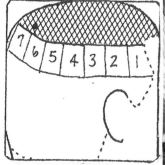
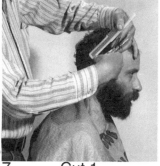
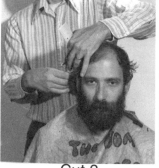
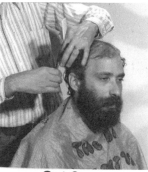

Path 1, cuts 1 through 7   Cut 1   Cut 2   Cut 3

To accommodate the back section and its 6 inch-long growing surface, use an equal-length positioning with your left hand as you do the rest of the path around the back.

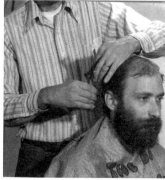
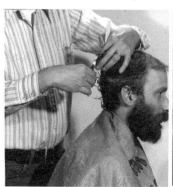
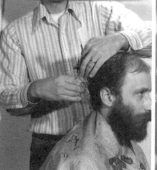
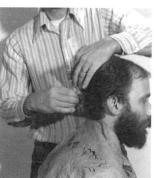

Cut 4   Cut 5   Cut 6   Cut 7

With a Type I hair grain, the sequence of cuts shown above works well. If you have a Type 2 grain to work with, you may have to reverse the sequence of cuts: start at the back of the head and continue to the front right side while using the comb-away method.

Remember, before you begin, comb the hair in the opposite direction from your travel through the path. Here the hair was combed toward the front before the cutting began.
Pathway 2 Again, the first three cuts are slightly tapered; then you resume an equal-length cutting for the rest of the path. Use the comb-away method. Type 2 hair grain may need the basic manipulation starting at the back and working your way to the front. The guide-hair from the top section is at the "V" of the holding fingers.

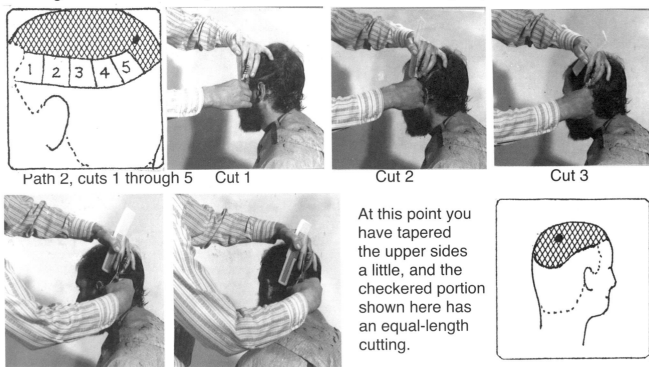

Path 2, cuts 1 through 5   Cut 1   Cut 2   Cut 3

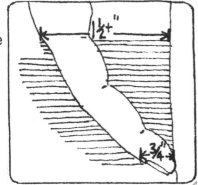

Cut 4   Cut 5

At this point you have tapered the upper sides a little, and the checkered portion shown here has an equal-length cutting.

Back to the right side for some "heavy duty" tapering:
Pathway 3 To do this cutting you manipulate your left hand as you did for 2-step tapering of neck hair (shown back on page 102).
Use the diagonal positioning, but now the holding finger tips touch the skin--this cutting is done to the hair beginning at the hairline and above, whereas the tapering you did on the neck hair was concerned with longer hairs 1 to 2 inches above the neck's edge line.Your finger tips can't touch the skin on the first cut because of the sideburn, but it can for the rest of the cuts. Your holding fingers curve away from the scalp, up to and including the cut hair from the first pathway on the right side--continue to use that guide-hair found at the "V".

Start at a 4 or 5 o'clock position and move to 9 or 10 o'clock as you work around the head. The pathway illustration is "distorted" to show all the cuts in this trip around the bottom.

***

Failures are divided into two classes: those who thought and never did, and those who did and never thought.
John Charles Salak

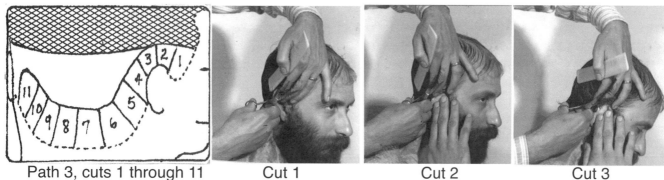

Path 3, cuts 1 through 11 | Cut 1 | Cut 2 | Cut 3

At about this point, you get away from the neighboring pathway approach as you continue down the neck and around the bottom of the back. There isn't any guide-hair to use, so be careful on the remaining cuts to keep the same out-and-away (curved) holding hand position that was used on the first three cuts.

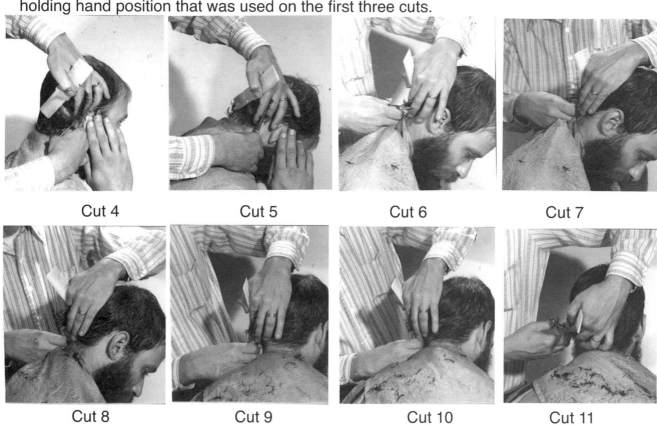

Cut 4 | Cut 5 | Cut 6 | Cut 7

Cut 8 | Cut 9 | Cut 10 | Cut 11

If the hair has a ducktail neckline and a strong Type 2 hair grain, this path may need to be started at the tail and travel around the bottom to the front right side, while using the comb-away method. Then return to the ducktail and do cuts 8 through 11 shown above.

Pathway 4 Cutting this path between the two already-cut paths around the back is the best way to get the long, gradual tapering that is needed for the back of the head.

You don't want this to happen.

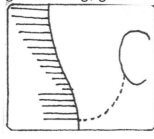

You want this--it's much easier to achieve when done as shown.

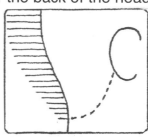

As these photos show, this path between the two cut paths has double guide hair to use (at the "V" and finger tips). Keep your holding fingers fairly straight, and cut all the hair between the two guides.

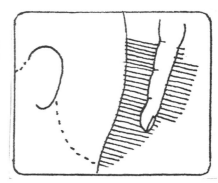

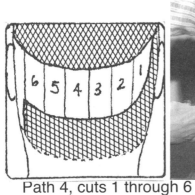

Path 4, cuts 1 through 6

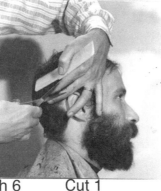

Cut 1

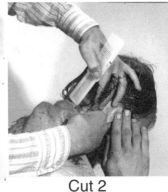

Cut 2

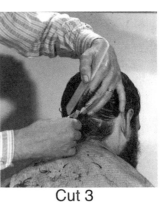

Cut 3

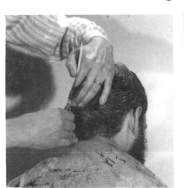

Cut 4

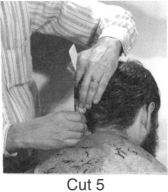

Cut 5

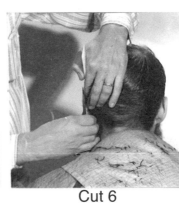

Cut 6

Depending on head and hand size, you may have to make an additional path above this one.

Pathway 5 This last path has you return to the "heavy" tapering given to the right side and back. The guide-hair is at the "V" again. Finger tips rest on the skin, at the hairline.

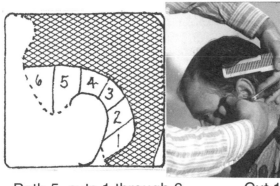

Path 5, cuts 1 through 6

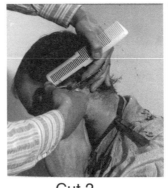

Cut 1

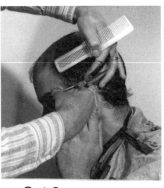

Cut 2

Cut 3

***

If you lend a friend money and never see him again, it's worth it.   Anonymous

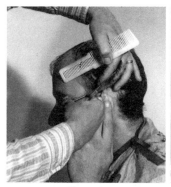

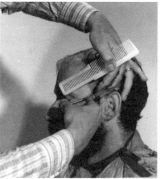

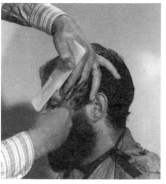

Cut 4   Cut 5   Cut 6

In cutting this path, it doesn't matter if the hair has Type 1 or 2 grain-this sequence of cuts works well with either.

9.3 SMOOTHING OFF

For this second-time-through cutting, go through the hair with the left hand held in an opposite position from what was used during the first-time-through. Here the holding fingers are positioned horizontally, instead of vertically or diagonally.

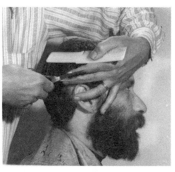

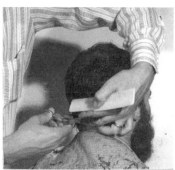

Before we start cutting, you should be aware of the following:
• The first-time-through bulk-removal usually leaves a little more unevenness than what you are used to, especially in this area on each side of the head:

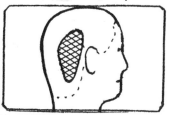

This unevenness is a result of going from the three-inch long sides to the six-inch long back section hair. This second-time-through cutting gets these areas smoothly-cut.

• For the second cutting, you start at the bottom of the sides and back, and move up through pathways from there. Because most of your tapering occurred on the bottom 2 - 3 inches around the head, each pathway up the head needs the stepping-out method (see page 103) for the first several manipulations you make up the path.
•How far away from the scalp the holding fingers are positioned for each manipulation is determined solely by the cutting done on the first-time-through bulk-removal. For example, the first cut in any pathway is always at the hairline: here your holding fingers touch the skin. They are in the shortest possible cutting position because the finger tips touched the skin when the first-time-through cutting was done on the bottom path.

***

Never in this world can hatred be stilled by hatred; it will be stilled only by non-hatred-- this is the law eternal.

Buddha

It is possible to live in peace.

Mohandas Gandhi

The hair between the holding fingers will look something like this:

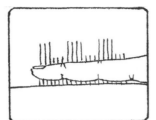

Cut off only the longer hair-- the shorter hair is your guide-hair.

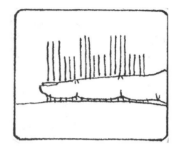

Because of the increasing length on the sides, when the next manipulation is made, one inch up from the first one, there is longer hair protruding from the holding fingers. To smooth off these hairs, slide your hand out on the hair so there is the same amount of guide-hair sticking out (1/8 to 1/4 inch) from the holding fingers as was shown above.

Cut off those longer hairs and your smooth it off goal is realized. When the stepping-out cuts are done this way, the cuts always conform to and blend with the tapering you achieved on the bulk-removal.

A. Sequence of Paths

1. Right side. The first pathway starts at the bottom of the front right side, near the sideburn, and proceeds up to the top-front center of the hairline.

Some manipulations will have you hold and cut small amounts of hair-- good. The idea is to establish a straight path for the next pathways to follow. Paths 2 and 3 are alongside the first path.

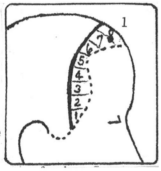
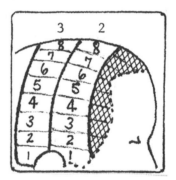

Stand at the 8 to 10:00 o'clock position for these first three paths. Have your chair in a low position and you'll need more than the usual amount of head-bending cooperation.

The next 2 pathways are on the side of the neck. These short paths are straight-away from the hairline. Stand at 6 or 7 o'clock and some ear folding help would be nice.

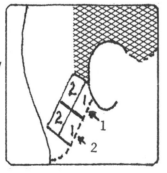
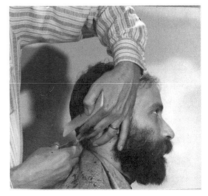

***

My belief is that to have no wants is divine.   Socrates

I am never bored anywhere: being bored is an insult to oneself.   Renard

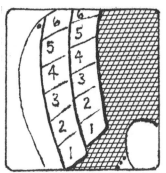

After you've finished the
the short paths, make two
paths up to the rear part of
the top of the head--they
begin where the two short
paths left off.

2. Back section. For the back of the head, follow the same pathways and sequence of cuts used during the bulk-removal on the equal-length cut (see page 92). The first path on this back section has you go back over part of the area you worked on during the side of the neck cutting. Good. This area is where most of the unevenness in a short, full cut is found--it can stand an extra going over.

3. Left side. The first two paths are the same as the paths on the right side, except now reverse the sequence of short paths, and the holding fingers point upward instead of downward. Keep standing at 4 or 5 o'clock for the two longer paths that go up to the top. (You're going over the last path from the back section--this area needs it.) Finish the smooth off efforts with the 3 front side paths, beginning where the last cutting left off.

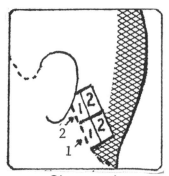
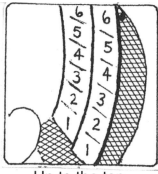
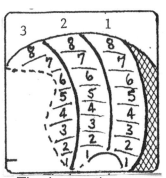

| Short paths | Up to the top | The last paths |

At this point, your precision-cut short, full haircut is almost completed. Before the edging, dry the hair and inspect it for heavy spots or cutting lines. Go through the trouble spots again, behind and above the ears--trim as needed.

9.4 EDGING

After the bulk-cutting for short haircuts (like the other two layered cuts), the edge-line is close to the way you want it. Just cutting a few stragglers is all that should be needed.

A. Sequence to Follow
1. <u>Bangs</u>. Because the top hair was cut to the same length, use the same methods here as used for the equal-length cut.
2. <u>Upper right temple region</u>. The questions of whether to trim and what methods to use are the same for this cut as for the equal-length cut (see page 110).

3. <u>Lower temple</u>. Because of the tapered cutting around the lower sides, the edging also has a decreasing length. Before you cut, comb the hair back to see the shape of the hairline. Then comb the hair toward the front and use the finger-bracing or the scissors-and-comb method (or both).

Give the lower temple region this kind of decreasing length on the edge line. This makes the edge cuts conform to the bulk-removal tapering.

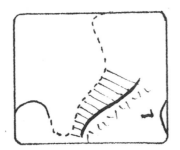

4. <u>Right sideburn</u>. Do this cutting the same as it was done on the equal-length haircut.
5. <u>Right side</u>. A short cut limits the edging methods that can be used because of the length of the hair. Comb the hair straight away from the hairline and use the finger-bracing method. On a Type 2 hair grain, the scissors-and-comb method may have to be used to get the hair straight out from the hair line--particularly above and behind the ear.

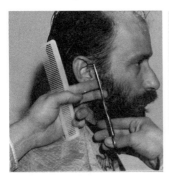
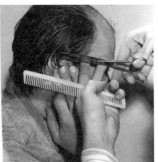
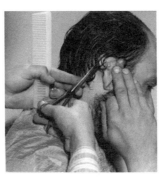

Any part of this edging may need you to reverse the direction the scissors takes. Do whatever is easiest and most effective.

On a Type 2 grain, the cutting path should begin at the bottom of the neck and go upward over the ear (page 145 explained why).
6. <u>Neckline.</u> Use the finger-bracing method to cut a line across the back. Be sure the line is at or below the hairline.

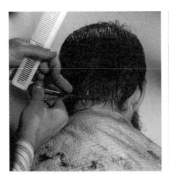
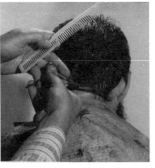
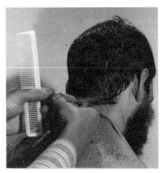

After you round off the corner where the right side of the neck and the bottom neckline meet, go to the left temple and work your way to the back on the "port" side.

After the finishing touches, you ll have produced another haircut that lives up to all claims of low maintenance, ignorable, healthy hair.

***

The reward for work well done is the opportunity to do more.   Jonas Salk

151

9.5 OTHER APPROACHES TO BULK-REMOVAL

When I work in my professional environment, I usually give a short, full cut by first cutting the upper two-thirds of the hair using the methods shown in the photos; for the bottom third, I use a clipper-over-comb cutting to get the hair tapered. (Page 174 has a short how-to). For me, with my experience, this is a quick and easy way to do it. But I find an all scissor and comb cutting, as shown here is needed in these situations:
• With little ones who are scared by the sound of the clippers.
• If I'm doing the cutting outdoors without access to electricity.
Eventually your skills will develop to the point where you can use the clipper-over-comb way to taper the lower portions of the sides and back. As a beginner, success is more easily achieved with the scissors-and-comb way to give short cuts. Besides choices of tools used, you may also choose a different cutting sequence for the short, full haircut:
1. After the top section has been cut, use the same stepping-out method around the sides and back that was recommended for the second-time-through part of the haircut. Doing it this way, the second-time cutting would require a vertical hand position around the sides and back, but the usual diagonal cutting around the bottom paths.
2. Again, after the top section is cut in the usual manner, do the back section by stepping-out (horizontal hand positioning). Then do the right and left sides with the vertical or diagonal hand positioning. For the second-time-through, use the vertical or diagonal position on the back, and horizontal stepping-out cuts on the sides.
3. For a little change, I sometimes do the edging first before any bulk-removal.

9.6 SHAPING OPTIONS WITH THE SHORT CUT

Short haircuts were my "bread and butter" throughout the 1960s. Since the late 60s longer cuts have taken over, but shorter cuts still make up a large percentage of my haircuts. Our survey of other ways to give short haircuts begins with a look at recent haircutting history.

A. Short Cuts Aren't So Short
Prior to the 1970s, just about all edging around the ears and down the sides of the neck was done as short and close to the natural hairline as possible. In addition, the bottom neck hair was usually tapered extra short.

A short "fresh-cut" approach at the neckline has this shape:

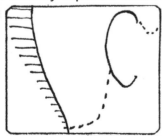

Short, full cuts are left longer on the bulk-removal, and the line cut across the bottom leaves extra fullness.

***

Men once subscribed to the theory of male superiority, but women have cancelled the subscription
Anonymous

Feminists just want the human race to be a tie.
Anonymous

An increasing number of folks want the edge line around the ears, neckline,and sideburn area left longer so the haircut appears a month old. The idea is to cut the edge hair so the cutting line is 1/2 or 3/4 inch away from the hairline.

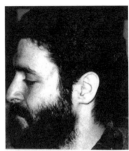

This "been worn awhile" way of cutting is very appropriate for those who are making a big change from a long haircut to one of these shorter cuts--it eases the transition.

With this edge line treatment, those extra neck hairs that are normally shaved or clipped off, should get a scissors-over-comb cutting that leaves them about 1/2 inch long.

B. Short, Full Cut with a Longer Top

Short, full cuts can be given to virtually any head of hair with excellent results. The major exception occurs with that rare person who has a troublesome double cowlick that stands up if cut to a length of 2 1/2 inches or shorter. If you encounter someone with a rooster tail from twin cowlicks, leave the top 3 - 3 1/2 inches long so there is enough extra length for the hair to bend into a lying position. This extra-length cutting will need some tapering done to the hair on pathways 4 and 5 on the top section. This tapering is done just on the upper sides--not on the cutting around the upper back of the head. With this extra length left on the top, you may have to cut off more than the minimum amount when edge-cutting the bangs.

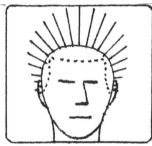 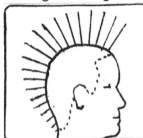 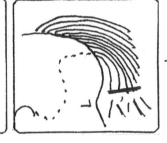 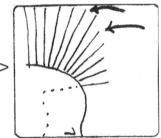

The arrows in the last illustration show the area that needs a little tapering after the bangs are cut. Take care of this with the second time-through cutting.

Besides being a good length for the stand-on-end double cowlick, this is the length to leave straight hair if the top hair is worn toward the back despite its natural inclinations to lie toward the front--it takes extra length for it to bend.

C. The Extra Full, Short Cut

With this kind of shaping there is extra length and fullness around the sides and back, instead of on top as the previous option had.

1. Bulk removal. Give an equal-length cut to the whole head of hair. The best length would be 2 or 2 1/2 inches; however, it can be cut as short as 1 1/2 inches or as long as 3 inches, depending on texture or hair type. If the hair around the bottom of the sides and back is shorter than the cutting length you have decided on,(from a previous haircut,) ignore those shorter hairs and go ahead and cut the rest of the hair to the

***

Generous people are rarely mentally ill.   Dr. Karl Menninger

desired length--those short ones get dealt with later. Taper the bottom neck hair using the stepping-out method while doing the bulk-removal.

2. Edging. Cut the bangs and temple region hair as it's done on the equal-length cut. The edging around the the ears depends on the hair grain there.

• Type 1 hair grain. Cut in the edge line the same way it was done on the regular short, full cut. However, to keep the extra fullness, do the edging away from the hairline--as close to the ear as possible.

• Type 2 hair grain. Cut the edge line in the ear are as you did for the equal-length cut.

Leave 1/2 to 1 inch of hair covering the top of the ear when the hair is combed straight down. When that hair is combed back, so it lies in its preferred position, it lies above the ear, creating extra fullness.

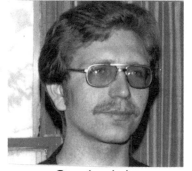 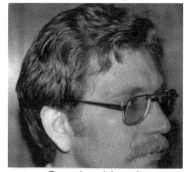

Combed down.   Combed back.

Do the edging down the sides of the neck as you did it for the equal-length cut. Because this cut has the neck hair tapered, your edge line toward the bottom of the side of the neck conforms to that tapered cutting.

3. A little tapering. Besides tapering the neck hair somewhat, the hair that covers the ear will probably need some too if you cut off an inch or more while doing the edging there.

D. Finger Cut

Because my hair is "as fine as frog's hair", plus a forehead that seems to grow every year, plus I have the short-growing hair problem around the lower sides, this is my haircut. (With all these hair conditions, I don't have much choice.) On this cut you're actually giving an equal-length cut, except that here there is no space between the scalp and the holding fingers-they lie flat on the scalp. Cutting off all the hair that protrudes above the holding fingers leaves the hair 3/4 to 1 inch long all over. Follow the same sequence of cuts used on the equal-length cut. This is the easiest of the short cuts to give--it's in this part of the chapter because its short length is not adaptable to many heads of hair.

This cut works especially well with soft, baby-fine, straight or wavy hair--the coarser varieties will stand on end if cut this short. When it comes to curly or kinky hair, it doesn't make any difference if the hair is baby-fine or as coarse as #14 wire: it lies in closely spaced waves or stands out in smoothly cut curls, even with the skinniest of holding fingers.

Except for the lower temple region, do all the edging as you did it for the short, full cut. The lower temple, because of the equal-length bulk-removal, needs to be cut with the edge line equal distance from the hairline.

The next chapter presents the "Bob" haircut--a big change from the layered approach to cutting hair.

CHAPTER 10 THE BOB HAIRCUT

10.1 INTRODUCTION

This shortest of the haircut chapters shows how to give a haircut that has been very popular with ladies since the 1920s. When my Dad began barbering in the late 1920s learning to give this haircut made the difference between an ample income and a skimpy one.. This haircut's popularity has to do with the long appearance of the haircut, that is actually cut quite short, especially in the back. This haircut is different from layered haircuts in that you do a little sectioning of the hair, and your cutting is done close to the neck, back and sides.

The layered haircuts have a variety of descriptive names including the "90 degree" for the equal-length cut, "180 degree" for the long-layered cut, and "45 degree" for the tapered short-full cut. Using this kind of terminology, the Bob could be termed the zero degree haircut.

Much less scissor work is done on this haircut, although a shorter version can get a scissor over comb tapering on the bottom neck hair--this kind of cutting has many "clicks" of the scissors as the comb travels up from the bottom neck hair.

10.2 SUITABLE HAIR

This haircut could be given to most any kind of hair, but as one who always checks out people's hair (the barber's curse) at least 90 percent of the Bobs I see are on straight hair, with the rest on slightly wavy hair. I haven't noticed a Bob on any woman with curly or kinky hair.

The Bob transforms long stringy-looking straight hair into a sharp hairdo that's easy to care for. Daily shampooing and brushing won't be a painful snarly experience the way it is when the hair was long.

10.3 THE CUTTING

This how-to shows a standard version with a couple of variations. Unlike layered haircuts, success on this haircut depends on your customer being able to bend their neck and head away from where you're doing the cutting. Expect to remind your customer from time to time about this. Here's how you go about it:

A. Before it's cut. The hair should be shampooed sometime during the day of the haircut. Begin by thoroughly wetting the hair with a spray bottle--it needs to be kept wet for the cutting . It's important to comb or brush out the hair so it has a **center part** on top with the sides and back lying straight down.

B. A little sectioning. A Bob with tapered neck hair doesn't need to be sectioned, but the standard bob is left longer so it needs this treatment for the back neck hair to lie well at the bottom. Sectioning needs a comb to part the hair and a pair of hair clips to hold the hair up and out of your way. Do a center part on top, and continue it down the back to the neck. Make two parts off to the sides, about two inches up from the neckline.

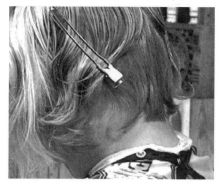

Comb the hair below the parts down.

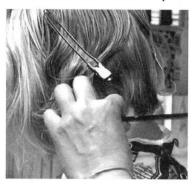

The clips hold the hair above the parts out of your way while the neck hair is cut.

C. Neck hairs get cut. The cutting begins with your customer's head positioned as far down as possible--if their chin rests on their chest, that's as good as it gets. They should **not** have their legs crossed--that can throw off your cutting line. Cut a line from the center of the neck (at or slightly below the neckline) over to the left side of the neck--use that as a guide as you cut over to the right side. This Bob has the cutting line straight across--a slight curve with the high point of the curve at the spine is common too.

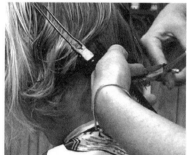

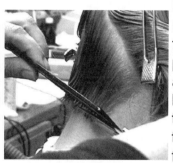

Next, repeat the parting, an inch higher than the first.

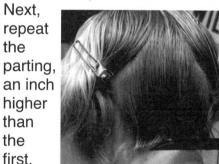

Pull and cut used here   Scissor and comb here

Do the same cutting, but now it's left a 1/4 inch lower than the first cutting.

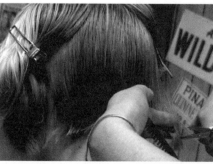

Because this second-time cutting covers over the first cutting, you need to go slow and look closely to see the cut hairs from the first cutting. Use those cut hairs as a guide for this cutting.

Repeat this parting and cutting the neckline slightly longer one or two more times--after that, if there are any back hairs long enough to reach down to your last cutting line, cut those hairs at the last line. If the neck hair doesn't have a severe ducktail, this way of cutting prevents (or at least minimizes) any flip out hairs at the bottom of the neck.

D. Cut the sides. I cut the right side first, but either side can be first. Begin by making a horizontal part on the side, an inch above the ear. Clip up the hair above the part so it's out of your way. Re-wet this side hair with a spray bottle.

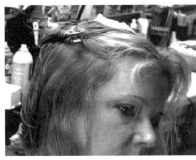
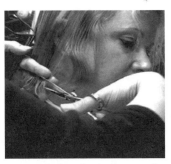
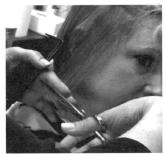

The cutting line continues the line used on the back.

Drop down the hair that was clipped up, and the hair from the top--follow the same cutting line, but like the back, cut it a quarter inch longer than the first cutting. Pay close attention to where the finished cutting line is in relation to the side of the face--repeat the same cutting line on the other side.

E. Edge cutting on the top. Now you comb all the top hair forward and down--the customer tilts their head forward somewhat. Cut the hair (which is now down below the chin) so those edge hairs are a continuation of the edge hairs established on the front side hair, closest to the face.

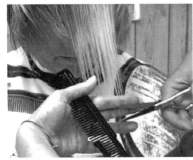
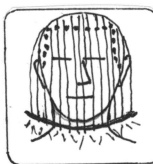
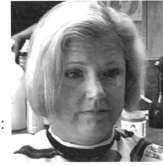

The heavy line is my cutting line.

After it's been cut, a nice result:

For cutting purposes, the hair on top needs to be parted in the center. This is important because if the Bob is cut with the hair parted on the side, the bottom edge hair on the part side will have long hairs mixed with the shorter edge hairs. Having long hairs show up at the bottom of the part side can't happen if the hair continues to get the exact same parting all the time; but hair doesn't usually get the **exact** same part every time, and hair can get mussed/windblown to cause longer hairs from the top to come down to the edges. If the hair gets a side part after being cut with the center part on top, no stray long hairs can appear mixed with the shorter edge hairs.

Bangs or not. Most Bob cuts are worn without bangs. Many have the kind of front hair that lies off onto the sides naturally--however, if the hair comes down and obstructs their vision, bangs will have to be cut or the front hair can be tucked behind the ears.

The tuck-in approach creates a kind of bangs, but the bottom edge is quite heavy, unlike the feathered bottom edge of cut bangs. Once the front hair is tucked behind the ear, the top hair (that's farther back from the front) will lay down the sides and cover over the tucked-back hair.

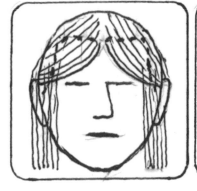
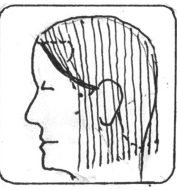

If they want bangs, it's fairly easy to do that, even if their hair needs a side part. Page 170 in the next chapter shows the how-to.

10.4 VARIATIONS

The Bob has many versions--describing a couple shows the range of what can be done.
A. The long Bob.
• A longer Bob can get the same cutting line on the back as the standard version. however leaving those neck hairs longer makes the overall length longer.
• A longer cutting is achieved by combing the side hair back and tucking it in behind the ear. This combing is done before the back is cut and is included in the back cutting.
• Instead of a straight across or slightly curved cutting, cut the neck hair in a fairly sharp downward curve.

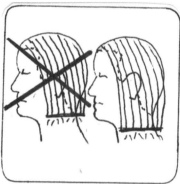
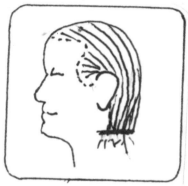
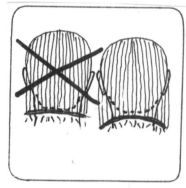

| Extra length | Tuck behind the ear | Sharper curve |

An extra long version could have the neck hair cut 3 to 4 inches below the hairline. This can result in the hair having the option of being worn with a miniature ponytail. Longer Bob cuts need a length check--see page 140 for the how-to.

B. **The short version.** On this Bob the lower ear shows and the back neck hair is tapered up to the longer hair that covers the upper ears. A shorter cutting like this is the best way to deal with an ornery ducktail neckline that can't lay down. This kind of cutting is adaptable to extra fine hair and to hair with a side part. The first two photos show the hair before it's cut, and the last two on the next page show the end result.

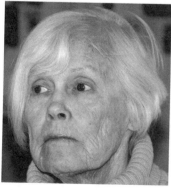
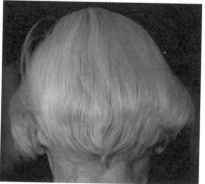
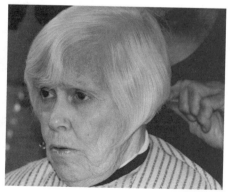

***

Compassion is not weakness, and concern for the unfortunate is not socialism.

Hubert H. Humphrey

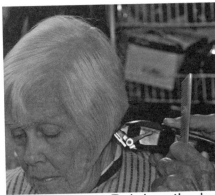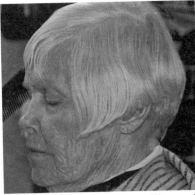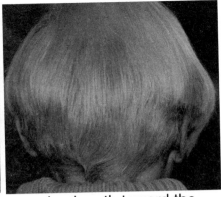

This shortest Bob has the bottom of the side hair with an increasing length toward the face. The short neck tapering was done with many "clicks" of the scissors over a comb-- a clipper over comb cutting could also be used (page 165 has the how-to for these tapering methods).

If past experience is a good predictor of tomorrow's haircuts, we can expect to see a wide variety of hair-dos come and go. The different cutting skills you've learned on the four basic haircuts will leave you well-equipped to handle any new haircut that comes along. Even though new ways of wearing hair are bound to appear, the haircuts that have remained popular have always been the ones with characteristics of practicality and simplicity. This being the case, it's quite likely that the Bob haircut and the different layered shingles-on-a-roof haircuts will be going strong as long as hair is cut!

The last chapter deals with a number of subjects that didn't seem to fit into any of the first ten chapters.

***

I am not the man I ought to be, nor am I the man I want to be, but thank God I am not the man I used to be.
Alcoholics Anonymous saying

Leo Buscaglia

The purpose of life is to help others

We are like onions, in layers. Many people live from the outer layer of the onion. They live in what other people think is the thing to do. They are merely imitative or conventional. Their conscience is that still small voice that tells them someone is looking. But we must try to find our True Conscience, our True Self, the very Center,... Here lies all originality, talent, honor, truthfulness, courage and cheerfulness. Here only lies the ability to choose the good and the grand, the true and the beautiful.
Brenda Ueland

Falling short of our culture's definition of physical beauty is good--you don't have to spend a big part of your life laboring under the notion that your skin and bone/muscle structure has made you a better person.
Anonymous

People should think things out fresh and not just accept conventional terms and the conventional way of doing things.
Buckminster Fuller

The real purpose of books is to trap the mind into doing its own thinking.
Christopher Morley

CHAPTER 11 SNIPS AND TIPS

11.1 CUTTING CHILDREN'S HAIR

Children need special handling to make their haircut experience fun and positive. Your efforts can result in a permanent customer who looks forward to having their hair cut, or something quite different. The following tips insure a happy outcome.

A.Their Hair and Its Needs

Children's hair usually starts out on the finer side, and slowly gets coarser until they reach puberty. This has consequences for you.

1. Frequent haircutting. The fine hair of childhood is inevitably weaker and much more prone to damage. Damaged hair = tangled hair = painful hair whenever it's groomed or shampooed = hair that usually doesn't get the kind of haircare it needs. Don't wait until the hair and its care becomes a painful drudgery. Instead, set a regular haircutting schedule of once every four to six weeks. When you give the haircuts taught in this book, just about all the ends are cut off. Those tangly, pain-causing ends are on the floor where they belong.

2. Delicate hair, scalp and feelings. Because finer hair is most affected by the many ways it can be damaged, the do's and don'ts should be closely followed. Pain-free hair is easy to have and it's every child's **right**.Their scalp is sensitive, so practice a light touch with your combing and as you hold the hair out from the scalp for cutting. Understand that first haircuts are scary events, so keep a soft pleasant voice to encourage the child's helpfulness. Remember, positive reinforcement always works much better than the alternative.

3. Cut children's hair on the shorter side. As Chapter 6 pointed out, if a head of fine hair is to hold a good shape all the time, with the recommended shampoo and towel-dry approach to haircare, it has to be cut shorter than larger-diameter hair. Cutting that limp, messy-prone hair shorter, gives it some body and fullness, and keeps it lying well no matter what's in the active child's day. Shorter lengths are also much less likely to tangle and snarl. As a child matures, accommodate your cutting to the hair's more coarse texture.

B. Safety Considerations

Usually a 3 or 4 year-old child is able to sit still and be helpful, but I've worked on one-year-olds who sat better than some adults. If you have a cooperative youngster, you won't have to do anything special. Those movers and shakers are a different story: they'll need out-of-the-ordinary tactics to do the job safely and quickly.

1. Kinds of haircuts to give. Because little ones are usually scared of the clipper's sound and vibration, first haircuts are best done with scissor and comb. With sudden movements a possibility, you lessen the chance of injury from the points of the scissors by not doing any finger-bracing edge cutting. If you have a "mover," you should give one of the longer layered cuts as these haircuts have the edge hairs in fairly good shape without any edging.

2. Time factor. You want to get done as quickly as possible when you work on a little one who can't sit still. You won't wear the child down, but they'll wear you down. You could give a short, full cut; however, you need to take extra care because the scissor is closer to the skin than on the other layered cuts. Also, the extra preciseness of this cut means it takes more time, and precise cutting is much harder to achieve on a "wiggler." Forgo any second-time-through cutting and accept less even cutting results.

C. Ways to Get Maximum Cooperation

1. Get the child used to it. For a few days before the haircut, the parent should spend some time getting the child used to the spray bottle, combing through the hair and holding the hair out from the scalp. You don't want any surprises on haircut day. Mom and Dad should avoid the term "haircut"--most children have been conditioned to avoid anything that "cuts." Instead use the word **"trim,"** as in, "We'll go to Barber Bob's place to get your hair trimmed." Another big help with words is to not bring up the notion of "tickle" during the haircut. That word only makes your efforts much more difficult as the child squirms away from any touch of your tools.

2. Timing can be crucial. From my experience, it's easiest to cut a child's hair right after they wake up from a nap when they always seem to be in a pleasant, fuzzy state that minimizes nervous energies and crankiness. Another timing issue that has an impact is to cut the child's hair *before* they have a visit to the doctor. A haircut is painless, but if it happens after they have been poked with a needle, they'il probably think they're in for more of the same.

3. At home. To avoid starting the haircut session with pain, the hair needs to be shampooed, dried and thoroughly **brushed out** so a comb can travel through the hair (all the way down to the scalp) without snags. If a haircut session begins with a painful comb-out, it's worst possible start before any cutting is done. This negative impression can be permanent.

***

Mankind owes to the child the best it has to give.   United Nations declaration

4. A faster option. If a child will sit still for it, clippers can be used **over the comb** around the edge hair. Use a very quiet clipper without showing it to them and they may not even know they've been "clipped."

5. Bring a helper or two.. Mom and/or Dad has a few important functions:

• **Keep the child's attention**. Little ones are usually very curious about that clicking sound they hear as you're snipping away. They turn their head this way and that to see what is going on--not very conducive to sitting still. Use whatever means possible (toys, a key chain, conversation, a T.V. with a VCR or DVD playing cartoons or a Disney movie like Bambi or Shrek) to keep their mind off what you're doing.

• **Get rid of the tickles**. Provide your helper with a hair duster, folded napkin, or wash cloth to keep those ticklish cut-hairs off the child's face and neck.

• **A lap for a chair**. It is hard for a child younger than 3 or 4 to sit alone on a chair or stool. In a short time, their back aches and they move around trying to get comfortable. Have Mom or Dad sit on the chair with the child seated on their knees. Face the child toward the parent and you have plenty of working room. You may be better off not to use a haircloth on children, because some don't like their hands and arms covered. Your helper can also help out by gently holding the child's head in a good position for you.

• **Extra help**. If it doesn't get too crowded, you may want two helpers: one holds and the other distracts and also keeps the hair off the child's sensitive skin.

11.2 BEARD TRIMMING

A. Facial Hair Options

The last few decades has brought a major change in the way men deal with their face hair. In the 1950s, a mustache was rare, a beard much rarer. Today a majority (or close to it) of men wear some form of facial hair. Many times a man will go through these growing stages before he is ready for full hair growth on the face.

1.Mustache.
Step one is to grow some hair on the upper lip. This growth may go just to the corners of the mouth or it may grow down a ways:

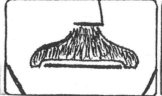
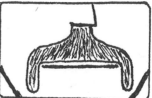

2. The goatee appears. This put-your-foot-in-the-water-before-you-jump-in facial hair comes in a variety of shapes.

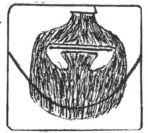
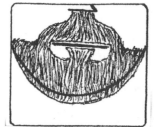
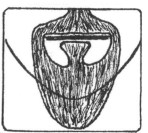

The bald spots on both sides of the lower lip are very common, but many men have solid hair growth below the lower lip.

***

Love for one's country which is not part of one's love for humanity is not love, but idolatrous worship.

Erich Fromm

3.Then comes the beard. The beard, like the goatee, can be cut and/or shaved into many different shapes. The following two approaches are the most common: they both need a fairly short (1/2 to 1 inch) equal-length cutting all over the growing area. The difference between the two depends on whether you choose to shave part of the face.
• Partial shaving. Shave the upper and/or lower portions of the beard. You normally shave in the edge line so that it is parallel to the jawline (the dotted line).

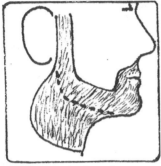
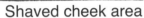
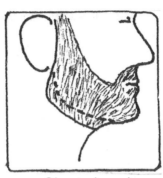
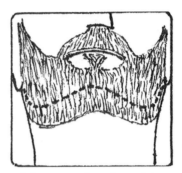

Shaved cheek area   Shaved neck   View under the chin

The main advantage of a beard is lost if some portion of it has to be shaved every day or two--perhaps that's why this next beard is so popular.
• The emancipated shaver. The most low-maintenance beard is the kind that gets an equal-length cut all over once every 2 to 6 weeks.

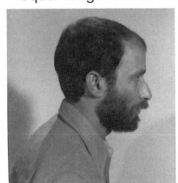
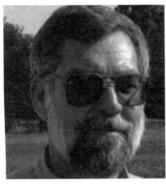
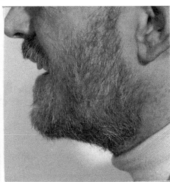

The majority of the beards I see (and the beard trimming I do) is of this type.

B. How to Trim the Beard: The Scissors-Over-Comb Way to Cut
Your cutting goal when you trim a partially shaved beard or no-shave beard, is a fairly short equal-length cut. In the barbershop I usually use a clipper-over-comb method of cutting. Sometimes I use the clipper with a spacer guide to give an old-time "butch" or "buzz" cut for the whiskers.

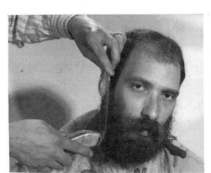
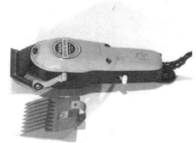
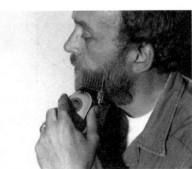

Clipper-over-comb   Tools for a "butch"   Using clipper and spacer

The same equal-length cutting results can be achieved by the scissors-over-comb cutting technique, but it does take longer. This cutting method has some new ways to use hands and tools. Here you keep the comb flat and equal distance from the skin as it travels through the beard. The scissors follow along, cutting the hair that protrudes from the comb. These are the specifics of this way of cutting:

1. Comb handling.

• Direct the comb through the hair, going against or sideways to the beard grain. The beard builds up at the comb's backbar, and you cut just in front of the backbar. This buildup has the hair standing straight out from the skin for the cutting, just as your left hand holds the hair out from the head during bulk-cutting. Here the comb is the spacer tool instead of your hand.

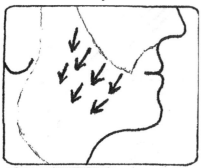
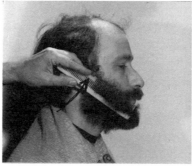
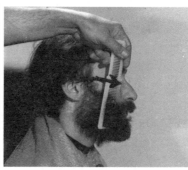

| Direction of grain | Comb goes this way | Or this way |

• Most important, you must maintain your comb at a consistent distance from the skin as it travels through the hair. The scissors cut only those hairs that protrude above the comb, so you need to pay close attention to the comb's distance from the skin. This is a bit more difficult when the comb passes over the curved areas of the jaw and chin-just go slowly and carefully manipulate the comb.

• Use the guide-hair aid from the paths you cut. The comb goes through the hair in paths that are alongside of paths that have just been cut. The shorter, already-cut ends (the guide-hair) appears at backbar, toward the comb's tip or near the handle.

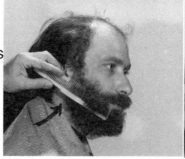
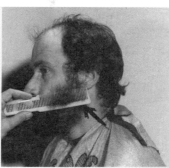

As usual, don't shorten any of the guide hair, but use them so the uncut hairs get cut to the same length. Use those helping hairs, but focus your primary attention on the comb's distance from the skin.

• The comb's thickness. The average comb is about 1/4 inch thick. If you hold the comb 1/4 inch away from the skin, you end up with a 1/2 inch beard length.

•Un-snagging the comb. When the comb travels against or sideways to the grain, it's easily snagged, especially when you start out through the hair. To get moving again, pivot the comb's backbar away from the skin 1/2 inch.

***

The five most worn-out words in the English language are: looks, want, get, buy and style.

Anonymous

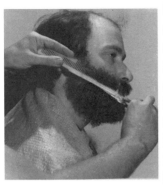

Slip the closed scissors under the comb, up to the snagged hairs. Remove the comb.

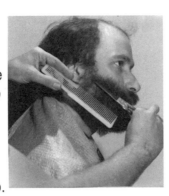

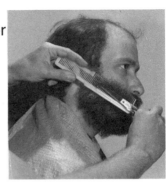

Reinsert comb under scissors. Reposition scissors at the backbar, and you're ready to move on.

2. Scissors handling.

As the photos on these pages show, the comb is the "director," setting up the hair and determining how much will be cut. The scissors are in a secondary role of just cutting the hair that the comb produces.

• Remember to cut a little in front of the comb's backbar. This is where the hair builds up and stands straight out from the scalp.

• Make a cut (an opening and closing of the scissor) for each 1/2 inch (or less) of the comb's travel through the hair.

• You open and then close the blades all the way while cutting. As you're doing this, you ensure a smoother, more even cutting if you open the blades fairly wide and cut with more of the center part of the blades. Short cuts at the points of the blades usually produces an uneven cutting.

• It's easier to keep the scissors cutting in front of the backbar when the thumb blade opens and closes, while the fingers blade is kept as stationary as you can.

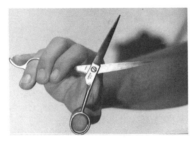

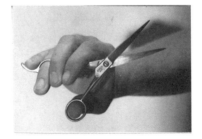

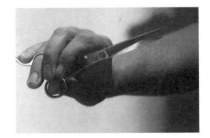

• Don't lean on the comb with your scissors as you cut. Hold the cutters so they lightly touch or are about 1/8 inch from the comb.

3. Practice.

You need to practice the scissors-over-comb method before you're clicking along without effort. Use the same practice I used in barber school: the rookie students would stand around a pole in the center of the school's shop area, clicking away with comb and scissors at imaginary hair growing from the pole. A goofy sight, but it got both hands working together. You can do your practice on a door jam. For more realism, find a beard wearer who doesn't care how short his beard is cut. If you botch things up, it won't matter if your cutting leaves the beard as short as 3/8 inch (the shortest it can be cut when you add the comb's thickness).

C. Tapering the Beard

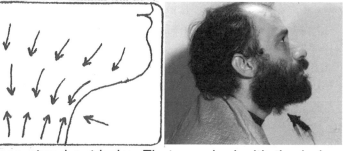

An equal-length cutting is the simplest and best way to trim beards. However, many men have a hair-grain clash in the lower neck area that makes the beard stand on end. A little tapering helps to keep this area in good shape. The tapering is done to the hair above those stand-out hairs. First you deal with the hair at the clash point and the hair below it.

1. Insert the comb a little above the standout hairs.

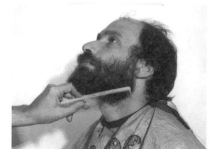

Comb downward while holding the comb flat against the skin. Cut the hair as short as possible (about 3/8 inch). It takes several paths to get all the lower hair cut.

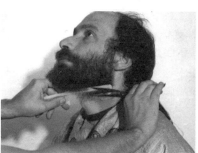

2. Start tapering the hair (above the clash point) where your short cutting on the lower neck began. Insert the comb into the hair, flat against the skin.

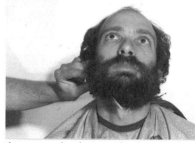

Then pivot the teeth of the comb out and away from the skin, while you maintain skin contact with the backbar:

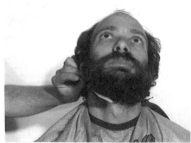

Move the comb through the hair toward the direction the teeth are pointing. The backbar loses contact with the skin as soon as the comb begins its trip through the hair, so be sure the comb travels in the same direction you establish in the beginning position.

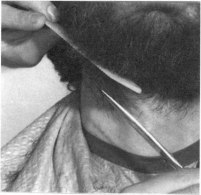
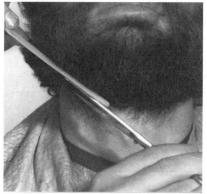
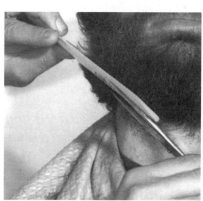

Beginning position   Halfway out   All the way out

(It doesn't look like it, but hair was being cut during the shooting of these photos--the timing was just a little off as the shutter snapped and the scissors closed.)

As with the short cutting on the lower neck hair, it takes several paths to get all the upper neck hair tapered. Be sure to use that guide hair after the first path.How far the teeth are pointed away from the skin when you first position the comb determines how gradual or abrupt the tapering is. If you pivot the teeth only 1/4 inch away from the skin, you'll have a longer, more gradual taper; 1/2 inch or more from the skin makes the taper fairly abrupt.

This way to taper hair can also be used around the bottom of a short, full cut or in place of the tapering methods shown for the equal-length cut's neck hair. Before using this cutting method on haircuts, you should stay with beard trimming until you have enough success to feel comfortable with it.

D. Miscellaneous Beard Tips

1. Length. The question of beard length is a matter of personal preference; however, most prefer their beard trimmed so it's a little shorter and has less fullness than their haircut. Most of my beard trims are in the 1/4 - 1/2 inch range. If you leave the whiskers longer than 1 inch, you could do the cutting with the same holding hand methods as used for haircutting.

2. Avoid harsh soap. While beard hair tends to be more coarse and less prone to damage, it can end up very tangly/snarly when bar soap is used to wash it. This problem is simple to avoid by using the same low-pH shampoo you use on your hair-- shampooing them together saves time and effort. (Low-pH cleanser is easy on skin too.)

3. The itchy grow-out. When a clean-shaven man starts to grow a beard, he can expect about 1 to 2 weeks of the "scratchy itchies." The reason why is not known, but it is a rare fellow who isn't affected by this distracting condition. You can minimize the problem by thoroughly washing the growing-out stubble several times a day. Other than this, all you can do is endure, with the sure knowledge that it's soon over. (It doesn't return when the beard is trimmed short, but it does if the beard is shaved and regrown.)

4. Mustache trimming. Beard trimming almost always includes having the mustache trimmed. A few things have to be cleared with your customer before any cutting is done:
1. Where do they want the bottom edge to be? In nine out of ten times they want the bottom to be right at the top of the pink of the lip. One in ten want some part (or all) of the pink covered.
2. Where do they want the sides of the mustache? If they wanted a "fu-manchu" type of mustache and you cut it even with the corner of the mouth, you've goofed.
3. Do they want some thickness cut shorter? Typically the mustache is cut to the same length as the beard, but you don't know until you ask.

11.3 HAIRCUTTING AROUND THE WORLD

While most of my haircutting has been to American Caucasians, being a barber in the U.S. has allowed me to give haircuts to people from all corners of the world and to all the major races. There are many exceptions to the generalizations I make here, but I'm confident these statements are a fairly accurate picture of the wide world of hair.

A. Southeast Asians and Native Americans
With rare exception, these people have black or graying hair, and it's almost always

straight with a coarser texture. Most (80 to 90 percent) have a Type 1 hair grain, and they don't experience baldness as much as Caucasians. All three basic haircuts work well. However, you should plan to give the longer versions with this kind of coarse hair.

B. Blacks

Black people's hair ranges from curly to extra kinky. Normally the texture is coarse, with many hairs per square inch. Baldness affects Blacks almost as much as Caucasians. The haircuts you have learned here are all very adaptable to this kind of hair. The equal-length cut, called the Afro or Fro, is the most popular of the three. Curly and kinky hair is easier to handle when using a large, heavy-duty comb. If the hair is extra hard to comb through, give it a hot oil treatment before the haircut..

Professionals who are experienced cutting Black people's hair usually use the freehand clipper-cutting method or the scissors-over-comb technique. Both are faster and easier ways to cut, but both, especially clipper-cutting, require much experience and skill.

C. Caucasians

A distinct difference exists between the hair qualities of Caucasians, depending on if they come from northern Europe, or the Mediterranean, Middle East, and North Africa.

1. Northerners.

• Redheads and brunettes abound, but most have blond hair, from darker blond to the nearly white blond.

• Hair texture is on the finer side, and they usually have straight or slightly wavy hair.

• With many exceptions, they usually have a Type 1 hair grain.

• Instead of total baldness, they tend to have a thinned-out hair loss.

2. Folks Around the Mediterranean.

• Brunette and especially black hair is the rule here.

• Hair texture is medium to coarse, and they usually have wavy or curly hair--the farther south you go, the curlier it gets.

• Type 2 hair grain on just about everyone.

• Hair loss tends to be complete, especially on the eastern and southern sides of the Mediterranean. On the western side, the Spanish and Portuguese are well known for minimal hair loss.

D. Other groups.

1. People from the subcontinent of India have hair similar to those who live around the Mediterranean. However, curly hair and hair loss is not as common

2. Canadians, for the most part, have the northern hair qualities of their English heritage, or the southern qualities of their French ancestors, or the characteristics of Native Americans.

3. Our Hispanic neighbors to the south have dark hair that ranges from straight to kinky depending on ancestry: Native American, Spanish, Portuguese, and Black. Type 2 hair grain prevails except for Native Americans, and the texture is on the coarser side. Baldness is not as common as it is for those in the more northern climes.

11.4 FOUR SEASONS HAIRCUTTING

This is a common-sense, ever-changing way of cutting and wearing hair that comes from living in an always-changing weather environment. Temperatures in Minnesota, range from 95 -100 hot humid degrees, to as cold as minus 50 or 60 degrees (when you figure the wind chill factor). With this wide-ranging temperature, hair can be an ally or an enemy, depending on how long or short it is. The weather-wise Minnesotan changes their haircut according to the temperature changes. A typical cutting cycle goes like this:

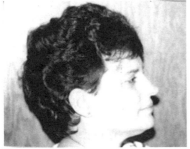

June: short, full
(top is extra full)

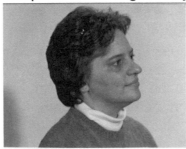

September: short
equal-length

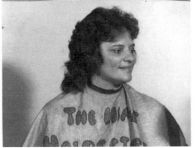

December: long, layered
(umbrella version)

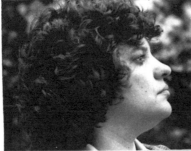

March:long equal-length

This practical-minded approach makes burdensome hair into a good thing to have around. Success with this kind of haircutting scheme depends on the kind of hair you have to work with, but you'll find a majority of your clients can enjoy this kind of flexibility. The only kinds of hair that won't fit into this weather related cutting routine are very fine straight hair, or problem hair that limits what can be done.

11.5 YOUR RESULTS WILL SURPRISE YOU

Cutting hair definitely is a funny and fun business. Many times, after giving my best effort while following the length and shaping rules laid out in chapter 6, I've had disappointing results. No, hair with problems didn't lie as well as I hoped; but, more times than not, that person came back for a second haircut, telling me their first haircut was the best they had ever received. These people have lived a long time with their problem hair, and have put up with a long string of poor haircuts. I always try hard, and the hair knowledge I've built up over the years (while it may not make a masterpiece out of a difficult head of hair), does maximize the hair's ability to lie well and look good. Over the years, I've built a large following of people with problem hair--they tend to be extra generous with word-of-mouth advertising.

Give the hair you're working on your best guess and best effort. More times than not you will do a very good job, probably much better than you think.

11.6 HAIR TYPE ISN'T ALWAYS WHAT IT APPEARS TO BE

Depending on length and haircare, hair can take on several different appearances. You

***

Commit random acts of kindness.   Bumper sticker

Racism is man's greatest threat to man--the maximum of hatred for a minimum of reason.
                                                                            Abraham Joshua Heschel

may think you have a particular type of hair to work on, but in fact, it is something quite different.

A. The Many Faces of Wavy Hair

• Cut wavy hair short enough (1 to 2 inches) and it takes on the appearance of straight hair that has ample body and fullness. This first photo shows a 2-inch equal-length cut.

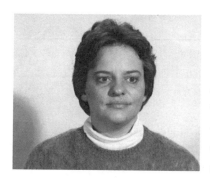

• When wavy hair gets long enough (2 or 3 inches) it's wavy again. Grow the hair another 3 to 5 inches, and it takes on a curly appearance. This photo was taken about four months after the one on the left, with no haircuts during that time.

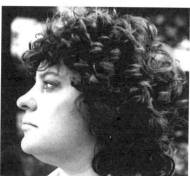

• When you grow wavy hair to a length of 10 - 12 inches or more, the weight plus the force of gravity pulls it straight, especially around the upper 2/3 of the hair.

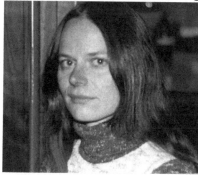

When you give hair like this a long, layered cut (in this case it got the umbrella version), some waviness returns because the extra weight is gone. If long hair is a little wavy like that on the left, it shows its waviness down around the bottom where there isn't any weight pulling on the hair.

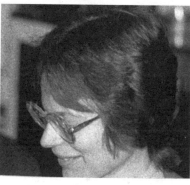

B. Straight Hair That Looks Wavy, Even a Little Curly.
If finer-textured straight hair, with a Type 2 hair grain, is grown long enough, the hair around the lower sides and back appears wavy or curly. This isn't because the hair has changed its hair type, it's due to weight and gravity causing the hair to bend downward, a direction that's contrary to the hair's natural way of laying. In this case, you're seeing *flippy* hair not wavy/curly hair, When that excess length and weight are cut off, the hair returns to its preferred way of laying, and the false waves or curls are gone.

Flippiness results when fine, straight hair with a Type 2 grain is grown to a length of 4 to 6 inches. The hair at that length ioften flips forward in the lower temple region. Cut it to a length of 2 or 3 inches, and it feathers back naturally.

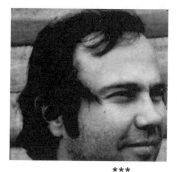
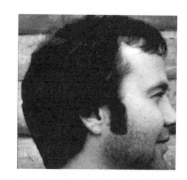

***

You may speak of love, tenderness and passion, but for real ecstasy discover you haven't lost your keys after all.

Anonymous

C. Curly Hair that Looks Wavy

If curly hair is cut to a length of 1 inch or less, it usually lies into waves. Let it grow another inch and it curls again.

D. Haircare's Impact

If you don't already have enough to deal with in solving this hair type puzzle, now add how the hair is cared for. How the hair is dried, and how often it is shampooed, will affect the hair's true nature.

• If you don't shampoo often enough, natural oil accumulation causes hairs to cling together. This condition makes straight hair appear wavy, wavy hair gets curly, and curly hair gets curlier (the same is true for the use of too much hairdressing). Infrequent shampooing means the hair also gets kinked up and bent from being slept on, giving a curlier appearance.

• When wavy hair is allowed to dry naturally, with towel-drying plus air-drying, or just air-drying, the wet hairs cling to their neighbors and wavy hair becomes curly, straight hair gets a little wavy, and so on. If the hair is drummed-dry, it lies much straighter.

11.7 TRIMMING BANGS

You already know how to trim the bangs for the different haircuts. Here you learn how to cut bangs when no other cutting is done. How you trim the bangs depends largely on how the hair has been cut in the past.

A. Growing Out the Layered Halrcuts

When any of the three layered haircuts are grown out, they eventually need some trimming to give the wearer an unobstructed view. Whether your cutting is confined to just bangs, or if it also includes the temple region hair, depends on how much the hair is to be grown out.

1. If you only want to remove a little vision-obscuring hair (instead of giving a complete haircut), all the hair that frames the face should be cut. This is necessary, especially on straighter hair, because temple hair falls forward into the corners of the eyes if it's left too long. The same edge cutting methods are used as when you gave the full haircut.

2. If the side hair is to be grown out for a time, but the bangs need some trimming, you need to avoid cutting the side hair.

This is done by combing the side hair down and toward the back of the head. Comb the bangs forward onto the forehead and trim.

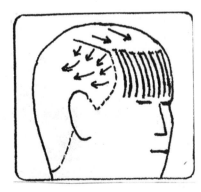

The bangs are usually left long enough to reach the temple hair-line that protrudes farthest toward the face:

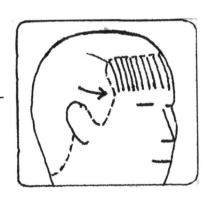

B. Trimming Bangs on Perimeter-Cut Halr

If you're working on a longer head of hair that's only had perimeter cuts in the past, your trim methods change a little, depending on the kind of perimeter cutting it's had.

1. Tree shape. If the hair's perimeter has been cut into a "tree" shape like it was on a long, layered cut, just repeat those edge-cutting methods (see page 131).

2. Bottom only. Creating bangs on long hair that has only had perimeter cutting around the bottom of the sides and back, requires special parting of the hair before the bangs are cut. How you do this parting depends on whether or not the top hair likes to part itself, and if it has a natural part, where the part is located--on the side or the center of the top. These are the two ways to do it:

• **The "V" part.** Use this part with a Type 1 hair grain that has the top hair growing forward (no natural part), or a Type 2 hair grain with a part at (or near) the center on top. You make a double part from the corners of the front hairline to a point back (usually 1 to 2 inches) from the center of the front hairline, thus forming an upside down "V".

The farther back the two parts meet, the heavier (more hair) the bangs will be. If the two parts meet close to the front hairline, the bangs have a wispy appearance.

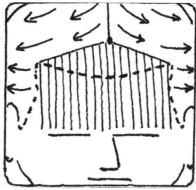 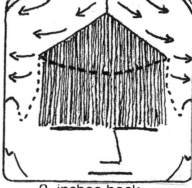

1 inch back   2 inches back

After you've made the "V" part, pin back the side hair and the long top hair behind the "V" parting with barrettes or bobby pins. Comb the hair within the "V" onto the forehead, and trim using the modified-bulk-removal edging method. If the bangs are going to lie forward on the forehead, follow the first edge-cutting with the finger-bracing method. This second edging is a minimum cutting that has you ignore the shape of the top front hairline as you cut the bangs straight across. If you want the bangs to lie somewhat downward and then off toward the side hair, trim the bangs so they are equal distance from the underlying hairline. On this cutting use just the modified-bulk-removal method, and leave the bangs with an extra 1 to 2 inches of length.

• **A side part**. When the top front hair wants to lie naturally toward one side or the other (with either hair grain type), the parting procedure for the bangs is changed. After determining which side the hair is to be parted. comb the long top hair to the side.

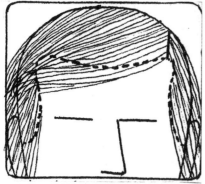

Then make a part that starts 1 to 2 inches behind the hairline on the part side. and goes over to the opposite corner at the hairline.

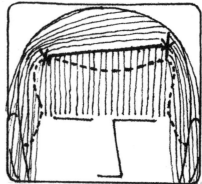

Again, pin the top and side hair out of your way. Trim the bangs as you did for "V" parting or use the modified-bulk-removal method and follow the shape of the hairline.

This type of bangs will swoop-off to the side with the rest of the top hair, so you need to do the cutting 1 to 2 inches longer than what you want for the final lying position.
The how-to descriptions for creating bangs also work for trimming existing bangs.

C. Variations

1. The edge line. Bangs can be cut straight across, conforming to the shape of the forehead's hairline, or with curved corners. The first two options don't need any more explanation; the third one does.

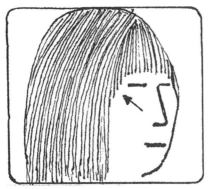

Pin the side and top hair back. Pinch the bangs into a single strand, and make one cut at the bridge of the nose (or higher). Follow up with a finger-bracing-the-scissors method to trim any stragglers.

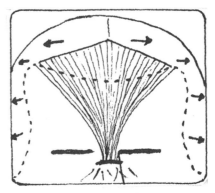

2. Soften the bottom of the bangs. If you want the bangs less heavy at the bottom, you can layer them a little. Cutting off 1/4 inch or less with the holding hand held in these approximate positions will do the trick. Each position shown is preceded by a comb-out.

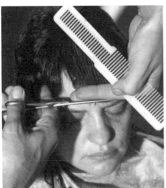
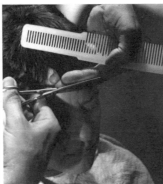
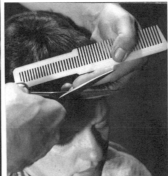
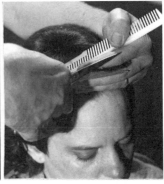

11.8 CUTTING YOUR OWN HAIR

Some years back I talked with a retired pastor. He told me haircutters and bartenders had the biggest opportunity to do some good for their fellow humans. According to him, we had the most time to spend in a one-to-one personal service that had the potential to be very positive. Maybe conversing while pouring alcohol for people does some good, but I'm sure constructive conversation and making hair nice to look at and easy to care for is, indeed, a very unique and positive personal service.. Because of this view, I can't get very enthusiastic about the do-it-to-yourself approach.

Besides losing the positive-service aspect of cutting someone's hair, cutting your own is quite a difficult task. Hard for all who attempt it, most find it an awkward process that takes too much effort for results that usually disappoint. Some people cut their own and do it well, but we'll never knowl how many disastrous cuttings they had to wear before they perfected their skills. Do-it-yourself cutting needs a mirror, and for the cutting around the back, it takes two mirrors. I feel a little awkward when I look in the mirror to trim the bottom of my mustache, so to use two mirrors would really confuse me.

Here a helper holds the mirror for the back cutting while the do-it-yourselfer looks in the mirror.

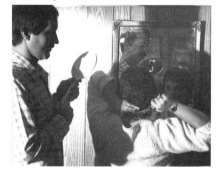

It looks like a good recipe for cutting the holding fingers. Go to a precision hair-cutter, and make make life easier on yourself and those fingers (appearance will show a major improvement too).

Trimming your beard is quite easy if you use a clipper with the spacer attachment. The scissors-over-comb method is a possibility, but like giving yourself a haircut, at best it's a slow awkward process.

11.9 HAIRCUTTER AS A MERCHANT OF CHANGE

Here we are, living in a universe of change. As a haircutter you fit into this ever-changing world because you create change. Every time you close the scissors on a handful of hairs, change happens. Because the majority of your haircuts are *trims*, (cutting just the hair that has grown out since the last haircut), the change made is not significant. However, on many first-time haircuts, you'll make notable changes by cutting the hair quite a bit shorter, or by giving it a different shape. You need to remember that people react differently to change--being able to "read" people on how they react to change, makes the difference between success and disappointing results.

A. People and Change: Four Categories.

People are referred to as individuals for good reasons. As such, I'm always leery of attempts to categorize people, yet my experience teaches me these four categories are fairly accurate descriptions of most people. At the risk of over-simplifying, this information is offered in the hope it helps you avoid people pitfalls.

1. The positive type. Given a good haircut that's easy to care for, these people are happy about the change that has happened to their hair. Typically, they are self-assured enough to handle any amount of change when it proves to be a better way. Almost a majority of my first-time customers are in this category.

2. The neutral type. About a fifth of the population could care less about the change a different haircut brings. They trust your abilities, and just want is to get it off. These functional-types probably won't want to see the mirror--they just appreciate being rid of burdensome hair. Don't be surprised later if they compliment you on your cutting skills.

3. The change-is-hard people. Another fifth of your first-timers are those whose initial reaction to their changed hair is something less than positive. They leave you feeling defeated after your best efforts have produced a haircut you know is well done. The thing to keep in mind is to give them time. The undeniable benefits of this kind of haircutting and haircare soon become obvious to them. In addition, they do listen to and are affected by the compliments they will get on their new haircut. Most of us have

some difficulty with change, but in this case a better way proves itself. In a short time, insecurities are forgotten, and your efforts are appreciated.

4. The white-knuckle, no~change folks. You could spend an hour giving someone the best haircut that person has ever had, and still have an unhappy customer on your hands. This small minority of people have a knee-jerk way of reacting to any kind of change--it's always "NO!" Even with compliments and the easy care advantages being obvious, the uptight ones won't accept what has happened to their hair, no matter how much time you give them. Luckily these people are a small percentage of the population, otherwise cutting hair would be a thankless way of spending time. This minority is even smaller as far as you're concerned, because their hair is so special to them, few would trust their hair needs to "just a barber," much less a beginner.

B. Avoiding People Problems

Going from a somewhat unsure, perhaps nervous beginner, to a veteran haircutter who enjoys the craft takes time and experience. As much as possible you should avoid the people in category 3 and 4. If you can't avoid them, at least understand the nature of change, and how people react to it--in other words, don't take their reactions personally. If possible, work your beginner's status off on the easy-to-get-along-with folks. Experience builds confidence, and soon your hands and tools are clicking along. At that point you're better able to handle the more difficult folks.

C. Making a Gradual Change

Many, if not most, people have some difficulty when a major change is made on their hair, even when they say that's what they want. You can minimize the change trauma by making a gradual change over several haircuts. For example, say you're giving a haircut to someone with the kind of long hair that has had perimeter cuts in the past. Over several months, you would make the first haircut a long, layered cut, later a fairly long equal-length cut, then a shorter equal-length, and then, if desired, one of the short cuts.

11.10 CLIPPER-OVER-COMB CUTTING

Video is, by far, the best way to teach clipper cutting. I realized this when writing a book on clipper cutting, and it's why I didn't finish writing that book. Various clipper-over-comb cutting methods are the heart of my "PRECISION CLIPPER CUTTING" series of videos. Whether it's video or printed page, these are the basics of this cutting method:

1.The tools. Use the same long-toothed comb used for scissors cutting, and any good-cutting clipper. The adjustable blade clipper shown on page 162 is excellent.

2. When it's used.This method can be used to taper the lower sides and back hair on a short, full haircut, the back neck hair on a short "Bob", and tapering the neck area of beards.(the beard section shows scissor-over-comb cutting, but using a clipper over the comb is faster and easier).

3. Dry hair. This cutting has to be done with the hair dry because wet hair doesn't feed into the blades very well--water softens the hair so it bends away from the blades.

4.The comb's function. Like it was with bulk cutting, the hair must stand out from the scalp while being cut. Scissors-over-comb cutting followed this rule and it applies to clipper-over-comb cutting as well. If a comb travels through the hair in the same direction as the hair grain, the hair won't stand out from its lie-down way of being. Insert the comb into the hair going against (or sideways to) the grain, and the hair stands out from its lie-down position, especially at the back bar of the comb. Whether its stationary or moving through the hair, careful positioning of the comb is the **key** to this way of cutting hair. Once you have the comb inserted into the hair, how far the teeth point away from the scalp is what determines how gradual or abrupt the taper is going to be.

5.Two ways of clipping. There are two ways of doing this kind of cutting:

•The comb is stationary. Here the comb is positioned in the hair with the tips of the teeth farther from the scalp than the backbar. The clipper moves to the left or right over the comb's surface **lightly** scraping the side of the comb's teeth, cutting off the hair that protrudes from the comb.

•Clipper and comb move together. This method has both the comb and clipper moving together as the two travel up through the hair. Like the first method, this way of cutting has the comb carefully positioned to start (teeth pointing away from the scalp.) If you were tapering the neck hair, the comb travels up through the hair, moving away from the scalp. The clipper follows along with the tips of the teeth cutting the hair that protrudes from the comb at the backbar. This method also needs a light touch with the clipper; don't push on the comb so it alters the comb's trip up through the hair

6.Keep cutting until you're out of the hair. With either way of doing the clipper cutting, keep cutting until the comb is out of the hair. On the stationary method, if a second or third cut is to be made higher up into the hair, position the comb with the same angle away from the scalp above the first cutting (now the backbar won't be in contact with the skin). Then hold the comb stationary as you make the next cutting across the comb.

Each time the comb is re-positioned for cutting higher up, the comb is farther away from the scalp, and it maintains the same angle as was established on the first cutting.

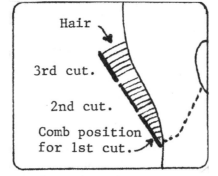

7. Guide-hair. As it was with scissors-over-comb cutting, do your cutting beside an already-cut area so you'll have some of that shorter cut hair at the tip of the comb or toward the handle, If more cuts are made higher up into the hair, you keep using the guide hair at the backbar or tip of the comb. Look closely to avoid cutting any guide hair.

11.11 DEALING W1TH PERMANENT HAIR LOSS

There are a wide variety of ways to deal with permanent hair loss. The possibilities range from the surgeon's scalpel to simple acceptance. This first option is the most expensive and least popular.

1. Hair Transplants. This is the Robin Hood approach where you take from the rich and give to the poor. In this procedure, an M.D. takes a "plug" of several growing hairs from the side or back of the head, and embeds it in the meager top. A number of these plugs, surgically transplanted, are an effective, long-lasting but not permanent solution to hair loss. The main drawbacks are the high cost ($20,000+) and pain.

2. Hairpiece. Back in 1972, suffering from a bad case of vanity/insecurity I bought a custom-made hairpiece for my easily sunburned dome. It took about a week before I got rid of it and accepted reality. From firsthand experience, I know a "rug" is:

• Expensive. At least $500 for a better quality version, and upwards of $20 a month for cleaning supplies and tape or glue.

• Uncomfortable. It is hot under that thing, and there is some discomfort in attaching it.

•Easy to spot. The sales pitch states you'll never notice a good one because it looks like the real thing. Baloney! Some are better than others, but I've never been surprised by someone wearing this cover-up.

3. The Big Flap

Millions of men try to compensate for their baldness or thinning top by growing hair long on one side, then combing that excess hair over their sparse dome. This is effective advertising to anyone with the slightest hair sense that the flap-wearer is in denial about a natural phenomenon. To attempt this folly, you must carefully part the long hair on the lower side.

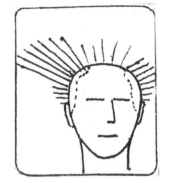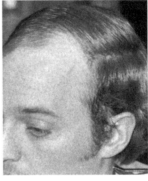

Some wear a few long strands over the top just for a laugh, but the big majority actually think they're pulling off some sort of deception. When the head is tilted forward or it's viewed from behind, that shiny scalp exposes their flimflam. Normal top hair also has some fullness; the flap lies flat on top. Long strands bunched together to resemble a front hairline is another sure sign.

This way of wearing hair has some negative health consequences:

• It needs plenty of time to get it to lie "just right," and more than a little time and concern to keep it that way throughout the day, especially on a windy day.

• Besides being burdensome, the flap takes away from the growing health of the surviving top hair. Because of the long-haired flap's weight, excessive bending occurs at the roots. Maybe worst of all, this hairy creation can't be touched in any way.

I give these haircuts from time to time, but only because I want to gain that fellow's trust so he might consider accepting his hair loss and my preferred way of dealing with it. To hint at a new approach to a first-time customer who has spent a good chunk of time and energy with the flap, will in most cases, blow him right out of the chair.

4. A Healthy Way to Make the Most of What You Have.
How people react to hair loss varies as much as night and day. Many cancer chemotherapy patients get so depressed over their unavoidable hair loss, they lose that fighting spirit needed to be a survivor. On the other hand, I saw two women on an interview program: both had alopecia universalis (total loss of hair), and for a variety of reasons, both expressed a genuine sense of liberation with their hairless condition. Many cling to their flaps and cover-ups as if the number of hairs on their heads was an important measure of their worth. Then there are others who feel hair loss just makes haircare easier.

 From my experience, most fellows already practice or are willing to try this relaxed approach that meets hair loss head on. Yes, it takes some self-assurance and acceptance of reality, but even the timid can appreciate the carefree nature of it, plus the healthy benefits. The haircutting how-to depends on the kind of hair loss.

1. Thinning hair. When the hair is in any stage of thinning, cut any of the layered haircuts as if you were working on a full head of hair. The only difference is to cut the top hair a little shorter (1/2 to 1 inch) than usual. Doing this adds extra fullness and will cover most domes as well, and in many cases, better than the long-haired flap. As you can imagine, a receding hairline or bald spot won't be hidden by the extra fullness: this is where acceptance is needed.

2. Total baldness on top. When the top gets to the shiny stage, and hair growth is limited to the horseshoe around the sides and back, you only need to follow the sequence of cuts for the sides and back with any of the three haircuts or their variations. If there are a few stragglers on top, give them a shorter equal-length cutting or cut them off by using the finger-bracing method close to the scalp, or you can even shave them.

11.12 MAKING A BIG CHANGE

Anytime you're making a significant change in the length of someone's hair--say 1 1/2 to 2 or more inches, you have some extra things to do to make it happen successfully. Assume you have asked the person how they wanted their hair cut and you have carefully analyzed the hair as to type, texture and hair grain (including problem areas.) You've talked over your analysis, and they agree on length and kind of cut. At this point, you need to get very specific about what you're going to be doing:

1. Before cutting, say: "So, I'll be cutting the top to a length of (for example) two inches, and around the the sides I will leave it full with a gradually decreasing length to about an inch long, and tapering a little shorter around the edges." While saying this you need to stand in front of them making eye contact and hold your hand so they can see it with thumb and first finger held apart indicating the lengths (two inches, one inch, etc.,) you will be leaving the hair on top and around the sides. This may seem excessively exacting, but I can guarantee you it's worthwhile--you'll avoid a surprised (and probably unhappy) customer by doing it as described.

2. Before or during the haircut you should be sure to communicate to them the notion that your analysis of their hair, while quite reliable in predicting a best length/shape for the hair, may not result in the *very* best length/shape on the first haircutting. In other words, you'll probably "hit the nail on the head," but if you're a little off, you won't be far off, and a second cutting will make the little modifications that will get you "on the mark." Haircutting is an art, not a science.

While I don't do it, I've always felt I would be justified in charging a little extra for haircuts that go beyond just trimming off the hair that has grown out from the last haircut. A first haircut requires extra time to analyze the hair and do the necessary communicating, and it does take extra time to deal with the longer length. In fact, it's a little like peeling off old wallpaper in that you have to work it off one layer at a time: First an approximate cutting, then the regular cutting, then the "fine tuning", then... It all takes extra time.

11.13 HAIRCUT RECORDS

Keeping track of how you cut someone's hair is easily done if you use my method. When I have someone's hair cut to their satisfaction I use a Polaroid camera to take a picture of the finished haircut, then write the particulars (kind of haircut, length it was left, problem areas, haircare suggestions, etc.,) at the bottom of the photo. With their name on top, it's filed in my index card file, and I'm ready for their next visit. By doing this, I don't have to go through a second "question and answer" session as to their hair desires. This method is also valuable for making changes or improvements on future haircuts: when they come back I ask how the last haircut was, and if they want if left longer or cut shorter, or shaped a little different. Knowing exactly what was done the first time makes it easy to modify the second cut to the changes they have in mind. Maybe your memory is good enough to avoid this, buy I deal with too many people to try to keep this information in mind. On the other hand, even if you don't need the reminders written at the bottom of the photo, it's nice to have a visual diary of your haircuts (and customers do appreciate this thoughtful service).

2012 UPDATE

In the late 1980s I changed my record keeping by putting the haircut particulars on the back of my business card. The returning customer hands it to me when they come for their haircut. This method worked very well for years, but sometimes technology comes up with a better way. This proved to be the case with the Apple I-Pad 2. This amazing little machine has a built-in camera and record-keeping ability. A better way came along, so we changed.

Any of these three recording methods work well, and are always appreciated by your customers.

11.14 THE LONG-HAIR TRIM

This is the last of the haircutting how-to. Cutting the bottom edges of long hair is so easy it didn't need more treatment than this short section. Yes, it is a simple haircut, but I'll point out some things that make your end product better.

1.Have the hair shampooed sometime during the day of the haircut. Brush out the hair.so it has a center part on top, and thoroughly wet it.

2. Have your customer bend their head forward so the chin touches their chest.

3. Typically, the back edge is cut straight across, but it can be cut into a rounded shape.

4. As you work your way over to the side hair, have them hold their head away from you. Cutting the side hair has you hold the hair to be cut somewhere on their shoulder or down on the upper arm. Be aware of where that cutting occurs so you can repeat it on the other side.

5. When both sides are cut, brush the top hair forward, and cut any long hairs between the bottom edges of the the two sides.

6. Check the length of the back hair by pinching a strand of hair behind each ear at the same spot, then pulling those strands together and down toward the spine. They should come together over the spine. If they meet to the left of the spine, the right side is longer than the left side, and needs to be cut shorter. If the strands meet to the right of the spine, the opposite is needed.

11.15 FOCUSED HAIRCUTTING

A focused kind of haircutting results in excellent haircuts, and a more enjoyable work day. Some things are necessary to do this kind of haircutting.

1. You spend time finding out what your customer has in mind for his or her hair.
2. You possess the cutting skills and quality tools.
3. You have the confidence to give customers what they want.
4. You know you'll be giving a very good haircut, but perfection is not attainable nor do you strive for it.
5. When you begin the haircut, check that the cutting is being done according to plan. Some haircuts start on top; after a few cutting paths up there, check if it is the length the customer had in mind. If the side was the starting point, check with them before moving on to the back or other side.

Once these things are taken care of, you can get into a zen-like focus on your cutting. This focus is a kind of meditation that has everything out of your mind other than the task at hand. Your customer may want to talk while you're cutting, but if you're like me, I recommend you stop cutting to do your communication (some can "multi-task" and have good conversation while cutting hair--I can't.) Resume your haircutting focus when your talking has finished. This kind of haircutting makes your 15 to 20 minute haircut fly by like it was 5 minutes or less.

11.16 CANCER DETECTION

As a 53-year cancer survivor, I admit to being sensitive on this subject (it was only a stroke of luck or ??? that kept me from an early grave at age 17). Prejudiced as I am, I always have my eye out for signs of skin cancer, and I also keep my ear out for things customers may say that suggests a change that could be trouble. For the things I may hear, I encourage them to go to their doctor for a checkup (what gave me a chance to survive). Skin cancer detection is something **WE** can do for our customers, and all it takes is to be a careful observer of the signs. First, you should know skin cancer is the most common cancer and early detection is the key to successful treatment.
Skin cancer has three types:
1. Melanoma. The rarest of the three is the most dangerous. In the U.S. in 2010, 120,000 cases were diagnosed, with nearly 9,000 deaths. These numbers are rising.
2. Basal-cell carcinoma. The most common skin cancer is rarely fatal, but it can be disfiguring if left untreated.
3. Squamous-cell carcinoma. This second most common skin cancer rarely spreads (metastasize) to the lymph nodes or other sites in the body, but it does happen more often than the basal cell variety.
Use the internet (Google: skin cancer) to see photos of the three types.
While giving a haircut, take a quick glance behind and on top of the ear, the top of the head and forehead (easier on a bald head), the back and sides of the neck and along the bridge of the nose. If something catches your eye, tell your customer about it and strongly recommend an early visit to the dermatologist or family doctor.
I have informed a number of customers of an abnormal looking skin condition that needed a professional look-see. For some it was the best tip they ever had. Those who got good news from the doctor have appreciated my being on the lookout.

***

There is nothing noble in being superior to other men, true nobility is being superior to your former self.

Anonymous

11.17 A PLEASANT, NO-STRESS WAY TO MAKE A LIVING

Before I wrap this book up, I want to put in a plug for the barber business.
Job satisfaction studies has barbering ranked at, or very near, the top of the many ways people spend their working lives. Based on my 50 year experience, here are some of the things I've found enjoyable:
1. Every 10 to 20 minutes of cutting produces a positive result. A smile and some kind words says it was job well done, and much appreciated.
2. My cutting efforts result in a haircut that make life a little easier. They are low-maintenance, low-concern, and require the least amount of resource-use to stay in shape all day.
3. Years of cutting has resulted in people who aren't "clients" or "customers," but good friends I look forward to seeing.
4. It's challenging work. There's plenty to deal with on the different haircuts I give, which are always customized to the person's preferences and the many attributes of their hair.
5. My shop is smoke-free, and no chemicals (hair spray, permanents, etc.) foul the air, or my lungs.
6. A variety of music plays without commercials, helping make a positive day go by nicely.
7. I'm free to set up and run my business the way I want. I don't spend time worrying about a lay-off notice. There is no age "discrimination"--as long as I can cut it, I can keep clipping away.
Success at this business doesn't matter what age you are; what kind of hours you work; whether you're self-employed at your own shop (costs less than $5,000 to get set up) or work for someone. All that's needed is a positive people-friendly approach and the ability to give nice haircuts.

11.18 IN CLOSING

Writing and then revising a book isn't like anything I've attempted before. The time it takes and the difficulties involved are much more than I expected. A few writing goals kept me plugging away. Slowly, but surely, I felt I was getting closer to these goals:
•Demystify the subject of hair and its care--what it is, how it's easily and healthfully cared for, and how to give well-done haircuts.
•Contribute to a kind of freedom that helps people avoid being concerned with the little threadlike things that grow out of the head. Showing how to cut and care for hair so it can be ignored throughout the day has been my contribution to healthy living.
•Make a contribution, however small, to the ecological movement. I believe there is beauty in simplicity when it comes to hair and that notion will contribute to physical and mental health, and to Mother Earth's health too.

HAVE FUN WITH YOUR HAIRCUTTING!

CAN'T FIND IT? LOOK THROUGH THE
CONTENTS LISTING AT THE BEGINNING OF
THE CHAPTERS.

***

**Knowledge is of two types: You possess it yourself,
or you know where to find it.**   Anonymous

MORE QUOTATIONS

When there were white spaces in the book, I filled them with words of wit and wisdom. Perhaps those quotations can be "fodder" for conversation that's not the usual weather, sports, and "how you doing?" topics. Of course humor is always good to pass along--a good laugh, even a chuckle or two is the best kind of medicine.

Printing a book like this is done on "signatures". Each signature has 16 pages of the book. Eleven signatures would have been 176 pages (not enough), so we had 12 signatures or 192 pages. With the opening pages, subject index, and another page describing my how-to videos, there are a total of 189 pages. I'm not going to waste three blank pages, so here's more good thoughts:

***

Christianity: Therefore all things whatsoever ye would that men should do to you, do ye even so to them: for this is the law of the prophets. Matthew, 7:12

Judaism: What is hateful to you, do not to your fellowmen. That is the entire law; all the rest is commentary. Talmud, Shabbat, 31a

Buddhism: Hurt not others in ways that you yourself would find hurtful. Udana-Varga, 5, 18

Confucianism: Surely it is the maxim of loving-kindness: Do not unto others that you would not have them do unto you. Analects, IS, 23

Taoism: Regard your neighbor's gain as your own gain and your neighbor's loss as your own loss. T'ai Shang Kan Ying P'ien

Zoroastrianism: That nature alone is good which refrains from doing unto another whatsoever is not good for itself. Dadistan-i-dinik 94, 5

Islam: No one of you is a believer until he desires for his brother that which he desires for himself. Sunnah

Brahmanism: This is the sum of all true righteousness: deal with others as thou wouldst thyself be dealt by. Do nothing to thy neighbor which thou wouldst not have him do to thee hereafter. The Mahabharata

Love thy neighbor as thyself. The Great Commandment

If these (the Golden Rule and Great Commandment) were followed out, then everything would instruct and arrange itself; then no law books nor courts nor judicial actions would be required; all things would quietly and simply be set to rights, for everyone's heart and conscience would guide him. Martin Luther

The test of our progress is not whether we add more to the abundance of those who have much; it is whether we provide enough for those who have too little. Franklin D. Roosevelt

The whiteman knows how to make everything but he does not know how to distribute it.

Sitting Bull

By virtue of being born to humanity, every human being has a right to the development and fulfillment of their potentialities as a human being.

Ashley Montagu

All that we send into the lives of others comes back into our own.

Edwin Markham

If we want to make something really superb of this planet, there is nothing whatever that can stop us.

Shepherd Mead

We have probed the earth, excavated it, burned it, ripped things from it, buried things in it, chopped down its forests, leveled its hills, muddied its waters and dirtied its air. That does not fit my definition of a good tenant. If we were here on a month-to-month basis, we would have been evicted long ago.

Rose Bird, Chief Justice of the California Supreme Court

The world is being run by (people) who really take no responsibility for future generations. And in this day and age, with science as it is, we have to be responsible or we won't survive.

Dr. Helen Caldicott

The world is composed of "takers" and "givers". The takers eat better, the givers sleep better.

Anonymous

We cannot hold a torch to light another's path without brightening our own.

Ben Sweetland

Life's arithmetic is funny; when you get to the end, what you have is what you have given away.

Anonymous

I expect to pass through life but once. If therefore, there be any kindness I can show, or any good thing I can do to any fellow being, let me do it now, and not defer or neglect it, as I shall not pass this way again.

William Penn

Freedom rings where opinions clash.

Anonymous

There are two ways to slide easily through life; to believe everything or to doubt everything; both ways save us from thinking.

A. Korzybski

Justifying a fault doubles it.

Anonymous

Every society honors its live conformists and its dead troublemakers.   Migno McLaughlin

We must have courage to bet on our ideas, to take the calculated risk, and to act. Everyday living requires courage if life is to be effective and bring happiness.   Maxwell Maltz

You may speak of love, tenderness and passion, but for real ecstasy discover you haven't lost your keys after all.

Anonymous

That man is a success who has lived well, laughed often and loved much; who has gained the respect of intelligent men and the love of children; who has filled his niche and accomplished his task; who leaves the world better than he found it, whether by an improved poppy, a perfect poem or a rescued soul; who never lacked appreciation of earth's beauty or failed to express it; who looked for the best in others and gave the best he had.
Robert Louis Stevenson

The five most overused words in the English language are looks, want, get, buy and style.
Anonymous

If one man calleth thee a donkey, pay him no mind; if two men calleth thee a donkey, get thee a saddle.
Anonymous

Children left unattended will be sold as slaves.
Sign in a diner

You know you're old when you've lost your marvels.
Merry Browne

Candor is a compliment; it implies equality. It is how true friends talk.
Peggy Noonan

Only YOU can prevent narcissism.
Bumper sticker

One of the symptoms of an approaching nervous breakdown is the belief that one's work is terribly important.
Bertrand Russell

Nothing will content him who is not content with a little.
Greek proverb

An expert is one who knows more and more about less and less.
Nicholas Murray Butler

In friendly conversation, someone's hair should never cause the other person to lose their train of thought.
Anonymous

Evolution isn't toward brains, it's toward sympathy, imagination and helpfulness. We are all on our way to be gods and goddesses. But we must help each other do it. Brenda Ueland

The measure of a man's real character is what he would do if he knew he never would be found out.
Thomas Babington Macaulay

The confrontation will be between those who are committed to making our presently inadequate social, economic, and political institutions equal to the task of repairing our ravaged environment against those whose first and enduring allegiance is to private profit and corporate power and the political institutions which stand guard to protect and preserve that profit and power.
The Progressive magazine

The best thing about the future is that it only comes one day at a time. Abraham Lincoln

Bad officials are elected by good citizens who do not vote.
George Jean Nathan

A person without a sense of humor is like a wagon without springs--jolted by every pebble in the road.
Heny Ward Beecher

The art of being wise is knowing what to overlook.
William James

Hell is not to love anymore.
George Bernanos

May you live all the days of your life.
Jonathon Swift

Suspect him most who trusts the least.
Anonymous

Think good thoughts.
Bumper sticker

Our life is frittered away by detail....Simplify, simplify.
Henry David Thoreau

If you realize you have enough, you are truly rich.
Lao-Tzu

Would a congress with adequate representation of women have allowed this country to reach the 1970s without a national health care system?
Bella Abzug

When health care is a human right we'll have a more just and civil society.
Anonymous

Parents can only give advice or put children on right paths, but the final forming of a person's character lies in their own hands.
Anne Frank

No one is happy all his life long.
Euripides

Don't talk unless you can improve the silence.
Vermont proverb

The past should be a springboard, not a hammock.
Ivern Ball

If it works, don't fix it.
Bumper sticker

It is the simple things of life that make living worth while; the sweet fundamental things such as love and duty, work and rest, and living close to nature.
Laura Ingalls Wilder

Some people see things as they are and ask why? I dream things never seen and ask why not.
George Bernard Shaw

Next time you think you're perfect, try walking on water.
Bumper sticker

If a man is alone in the forest and speaks, and there is no woman to hear him, is he still wrong?
Sign in a diner

***

MORE HOW-TO

Before adding photos and illustrations to a book I had finished writing on clipper haircutting, I realized **video was a better way** to teach the different precise movements of the clipper and comb. In the last ten years I've put together six videos: four were my own, and two had important help from my daughter and from a barber school instructor.

Like the book, the videos are sold with a "you're HAPPY or your money back" guarantee. Videos and the book can be purchased at our website: www.howtocuthair.com Sample videos can be viewed at our website, or they can be seen on YouTube.com--just type in my name.

...Bob Ohnstad

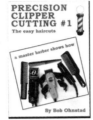

The first video was **"PRECISION CLIPPER CUTTING #1** The Easy Haircuts"   1 1/2 hours $27.50

They're easy to give, but precision cutting is needed for people-pleasing results. The fast, easy way to give Buzz cuts, Ivy League styles and basic Fade cuts are covered in-depth. Tool care and handling, including fixes for problems.

The next video clearly shows the how-to for tapered haircuts of all kinds. Includes analyzing the hair and dealing with hair problems. Learn the fastest ways of doing it, and get great results.

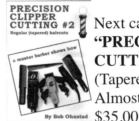

Next came **"PRECISION CLIPPER CUTTING #2** Regular (Tapered) Haircuts" Almost two hours. $35.00

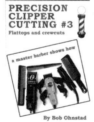

The third video was **"PRECISION CLIPPER CUTTING #3** Flattops and Crewcuts" One hour, 20 minutes. $45.00

You can give beautiful Flattops and Crewcuts with the how-to shown here. They're extra precise, but you're shown how to get great results every time. No guesswork after watching this video!

This how-to gem is a composite of the first three videos--same basic people-pleasing styles, but given to different people than were on the 1,2,3 series. When you know HOW, it gets fun!

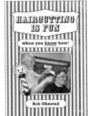

The fourth was **"HAIRCUTTING IS FUN** When You Know How" Two hours. $40.00

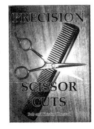

The fifth was **"PRECISION SCISSOR CUTTING"** co-authored with my daughter Kristin Two hours. $35.00

All kinds of scissor-cut styles, from the long to the short, and most everything in between. Cut it faster, cut it easier, and always produce excellent haircuts. Layered cuts, long hair trims, bob cuts and more.

The primary author is a barber college instructor showing how to give today's most popular cuts-- the Bald fade, Brush fade, Taper cut, and Tapered Afro. Plus beard trimming and best tools to use.

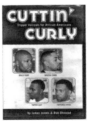

Our latest video is **"CUTTIN' CURLY** Clipper Haircuts For African-Americans 1 1/2 + hours $40.00

The videos include a **"cheat sheet"**--a helpful how-to reminder to use when doing the cutting.